HEART DISEASE AND HEALTH

HEART DISEASE AND HEALTH

Dr. Girish Gadkari

Jeffrey R. Larsen

MERCURY LEARNING AND INFORMATION

Dulles, Virginia | Boston, Massachusetts | New Delhi

Publisher: David Pallai
MERCURY LEARNING AND INFORMATION
22841 Quicksilver Drive
Dulles, VA 20166
info@merclearning.com
www.merclearning.com
1-800-758-3756

This book is printed on acid-free paper.

Dr. Girish Gadkari and Jeffrey R. Larsen. *Heart Disease and Health.*
ISBN: 978-1-937585-90-7

Library of Congress Control Number: 2012949960

121314321

Printed in the United States of America

Our titles are available for adoption, license, or bulk purchase by associations, universities, corporations, etc.
For additional information, please contact the Customer Service Dept. at 1-800-758-3756 (toll free) or info@merclearning.com

Contents

PART THREE Symptoms and Diagnosis of Heart Disease and Treatment of a Heart Attack

CHAPTER 11 *Symptoms of Heart Disease*

CHAPTER 12 *Diagnosis of Heart Disease*

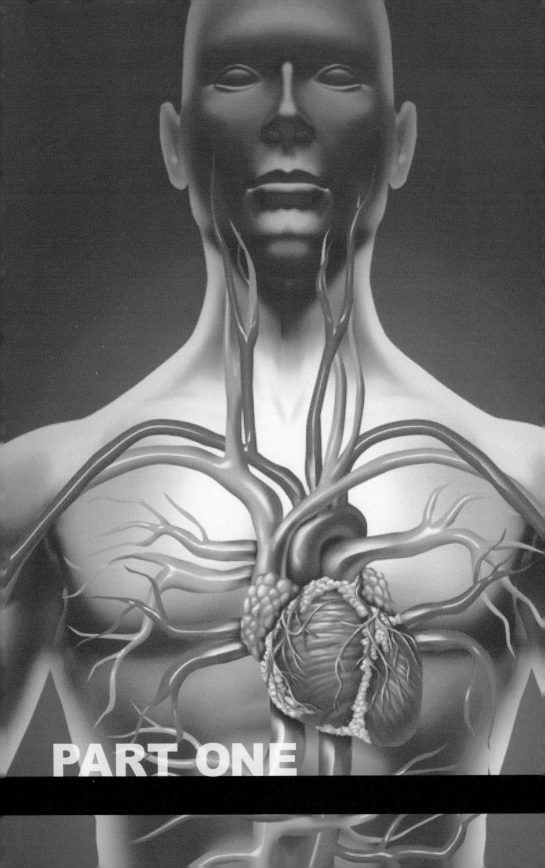

PART ONE

The Heart and Cardiovascular System

In Part One, we answer questions about the structure and components of the heart, and how blood moves through them. We then expand our discussion to the cardiovascular system and its role in the body, with particular emphasis on the arteries that are critical to the heart. Finally, we take a close look at the main components of blood and how they support essential functions of the body's metabolism.

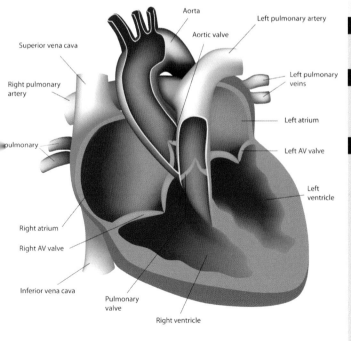

Aorta

Left pulmonary artery

Aortic valve

Superior vena cava

Left pulmonary veins

Right pulmonary artery

Left atrium

pulmonary

Left AV valve

Left ventricle

Right atrium

Right AV valve

Inferior vena cava

Pulmonary valve

Right ventricle

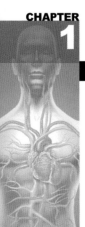

CHAPTER 1

The Heart

1. What is the heart and how does it work?

The **heart** is a mostly hollow organ made of muscle (*myocardium*) and connective tissue that performs the vital role of pumping blood through your body.

DEFINITION

Blood carries oxygen and nutrients that are essential for the proper functioning of every organ, muscle, tissue, and metabolic process of the body. The heart is located in the chest (*thoracic cavity*) between the lungs and behind the breastbone (*sternum*). The adult heart is often described as shaped like an upside down cone, and is about 5 inches long, 3½ inches wide, and 2½ inches thick. It typically weighs between 9 and 12 ounces, and is covered by a protective membrane called the *pericardium*. The heart is

The average adult heart rate is about 72 beats per minute, or almost 38 million beats per year!

NOTE

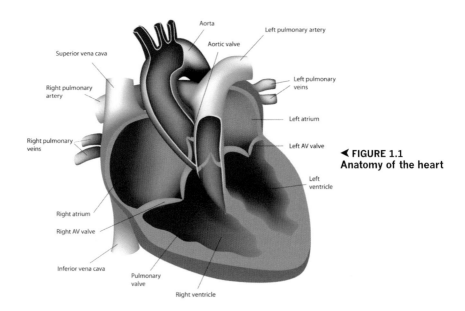

◄ **FIGURE 1.1**
Anatomy of the heart

Aorta
Left pulmonary artery
Aortic valve
Superior vena cava
Right pulmonary artery
Left pulmonary veins
Right pulmonary veins
Left atrium
Left AV valve
Left ventricle
Right atrium
Right AV valve
Inferior vena cava
Pulmonary valve
Right ventricle

divided into four cavities, or *chambers*, each of which serves a different function. The four chambers of the heart are the *right atrium*, *left atrium*, *right ventricle*, and *left ventricle*. The chambers are separated by walls of tissue and *valves* that open and close to ensure that blood moves through the chambers only in the proper direction. Because the heart is primarily muscle tissue, it is capable of the contractions—your heartbeat—that move blood through the chambers of the heart and eventually through your body.

The right atrium receives blood from the body through two large veins, one from the upper body (the *superior vena cava*) and one from the lower body (the *inferior vena cava*). Blood flows from the right atrium to the right ventricle through the *tricuspid valve*, and then from the

▼ FIGURE 1.2
Flow of blood through the heart

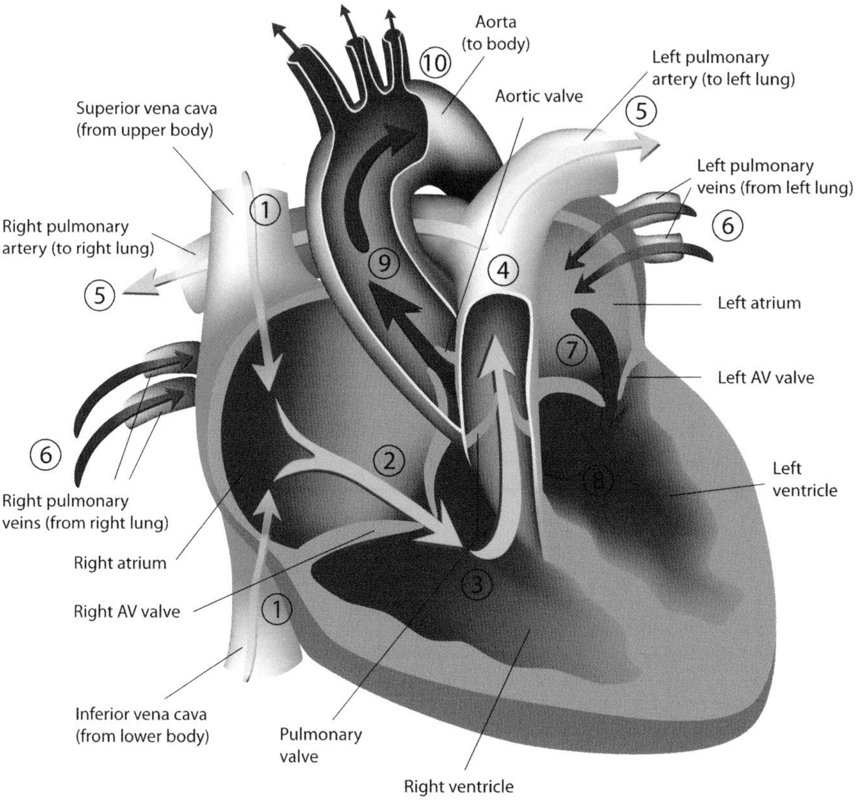

For an animated look at blood flow through the heart, visit:

http://www.youtube.com/watch?v=NF68qhyfcoM&feature=related

ON THE WEB

right ventricle through the *pulmonary valve* and the *pulmonary artery* to the lungs where the blood receives oxygen from the lungs and carbon dioxide is removed from the blood. Freshly oxygenated blood re-enters the heart through the *pulmonary vein* into the left atrium, and then moves through the *mitral valve* to the left ventricle where it is pumped through the *aortic valve* to the *aorta*—your main artery—for circulation throughout the body. To summarize the flow of blood through the heart:

right atrium > tricuspid valve > right ventricle > pulmonary valve > pulmonary artery > lungs > pulmonary vein > left atrium > mitral valve > left ventricle > aortic valve > aorta > rest of body.

The Cardiovascular System

CHAPTER 2

2. What is the cardiovascular system?

The **cardiovascular system** is made up of the heart, blood, and blood vessels.

i
DEFINITION

For our purposes, we can also think of it as the circulatory system—moving the blood through a network of increasingly smaller blood vessels that allow the blood to carry oxygen and other nutrients to all parts of the body. Circulating blood carries away carbon dioxide and waste products for disposal through organs such as the

NOTE

We noted in Question 1 the two primary exceptions to this general rule—the pulmonary artery carries oxygen-depleted blood to the lungs, and the pulmonary vein carries freshly oxygenated blood from the lungs to the heart.

lungs, kidneys, and liver. The circulatory system also helps to fight disease, and to stabilize body temperature and pH (the level of acidity). In general, arteries carry oxygen- and nutrient-rich blood to the various parts of the body, and veins carry away the oxygen-depleted blood and waste products.

Recall that blood leaves the heart through the aorta, the largest artery in the body. The aorta branches out to the body's main arteries, which further branch out to smaller blood vessels called *arterioles*, and from the arterioles, blood moves through the smallest vessels, the *capillaries*.

3. What are the coronary arteries?

The heart is a muscle that is always working, and it is surrounded by a critical network of blood vessels called the coronary arteries that supplies its oxygen and nutrients. The coronary arteries descend from the aorta and supply blood to the atria, ventricles, and other parts of the heart. Any coronary artery disorder or disease can have a serious effect on the heart when there is a reduction in the flow of oxygen and nutrients to the heart, and can lead to impaired heart function or a heart attack. The most common form of coronary artery disease is *atherosclerosis*, which will be discussed in detail in Chapter 4.

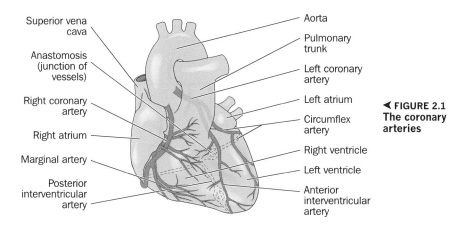

Superior vena cava

Anastomosis (junction of vessels)

Right coronary artery

Right atrium

Marginal artery

Posterior interventricular artery

Aorta

Pulmonary trunk

Left coronary artery

Left atrium

Circumflex artery

Right ventricle

Left ventricle

Anterior interventricular artery

◀ FIGURE 2.1
The coronary arteries

Blood is distributed throughout the body after leaving the heart through the aorta by the arteries that deliver fresh blood, and returns to the heart and lungs through the veins. Many major organs in the body have a dedicated network of arteries and veins to ensure their proper function. It is generally through the capillaries that blood transfers oxygen and nutrients into body tissues, and takes away carbon dioxide and waste from the tissues. Some capillaries are so small that red blood cells—the blood cells that carry oxygen—can flow through the capillary only one cell at a time. Depending on their requirements for oxygen and other nutrients, different body tissues have different numbers of capillaries. Tissues that have a high demand for oxygen, such as muscle, have an extensive network of capillaries, while tissues with little or no demand for oxygen—such as the cornea of the eye—may have few or no capillaries.

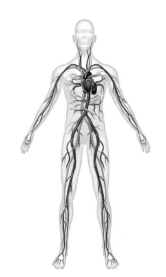

▲ FIGURE 2.2
The cardiovascular system

While estimates vary, it is thought that the total length of all of the capillaries in the human body could exceed 50,000 miles!

NOTE

In addition to the basic function of moving blood throughout the body for the healthy growth and maintenance of the countless metabolic body functions, the cardiovascular system can also respond to specific needs and conditions in the body. The smaller blood vessels—arterioles and capillaries—regulate the flow of blood to tissues and organs in response to specific stimuli. For example, when the body is cold, the arterioles that supply blood to the skin will constrict in order to reduce blood flow to the skin. This helps to prevent the loss of body heat through the skin. Similarly, after a large meal the arterioles that supply blood to the digestive system expand—allowing greater blood flow to facilitate the work of the organs involved in the digestive process.

Blood

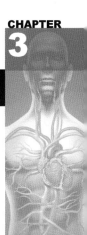

5. What are the components of blood and what do they do?

Blood is made up of four primary components—*plasma, red blood cells, white blood cells*, and *platelets*—that:

1. Carry the essential nutrients to each part of the body,

2. Remove and transport carbon dioxide and other waste produced by normal metabolic activity, and

3. Fight infection and repair damage to our body. Blood constitutes approximately 8–10% of human body weight.

Plasma is a clear liquid protein and saline solution that is about 95% water and makes up about 55% of our blood's volume. Plasma is the medium that carries the red cells, white cells, platelets, and metabolic waste through the vascular system, as well as carrying blood clotting factors, hormones, antibodies, enzymes, and important nutrients such as glucose (sugar), protein, lipids (fats), vitamins, and minerals.

Red blood cells (*erythrocytes*) are relatively large cells whose primary function is to transport oxygen from the lungs to all tissues in the body

PRACTICAL TIP

Red blood cells make up slightly less than half of our blood volume and survive for 100–120 days before they are removed from the body and replaced with new cells.

Watch red blood cells moving through a blood vessel!

http://footage.shutterstock.com/clip-180880-stock-footage-movement-of-blood-cells-in-blood-vessel.html

ON THE DVD

and to carry away carbon dioxide. Red blood cells are continuously produced in the bone marrow, and unlike most cells in the body, they have no nucleus. This is because they need all possible room to hold a protein molecule called **hemoglobin** that makes up 95% of each red blood cell. Hemoglobin is a gas-binding molecule to which oxygen and carbon dioxide attach for transport, and which gives blood its red color. A deficiency in healthy red blood cells, called *anemia*, causes a number of adverse health effects because of the diminished supply of oxygen throughout the body.

White blood cells (*leukocytes*) are a group of cells also produced in the bone marrow and play a major role in the body's immune system and cleansing the blood. For example, *lymphocytes* control the antibody and immune response by identifying and bonding to disease-causing cells and enabling other types of white blood cells, such as *granulocytes* and *microphages*, to surround and destroy bacteria, viruses, fungi, or other parasites. White blood cells also remove dead or dying red blood cells. There are many different types and sub-types of white blood cells, but together they make up only about 1% of our blood. White blood cells survive for only 18–36 hours before they are removed and replaced.

Platelets (*thrombocytes*) are the cells that facilitate the clotting of the blood by adhering to the walls of blood vessels and by releasing coagulating agents that cause blood to clot, thereby "plugging" any rupture or other damage to the blood vessel. The biochemistry of the clotting process is complex, and there are more than a dozen other factors involved in the blood clotting mechanism. Recent research suggests that platelets also play a role in the immune response by releasing proteins that kill harmful bacteria and other microorganisms. Platelets are formed in the stem cells of bone marrow, are about 1/3 the size of red blood cells, and survive for 9–10 days.

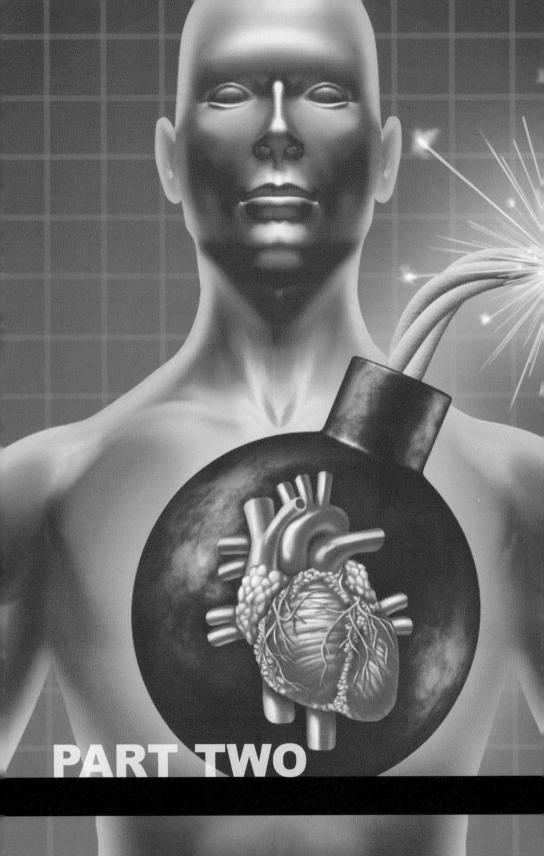

PART TWO

Causes, Effects, and Risk Factors for Heart Disease

After seeing how the heart and cardiovascular system work in Part One, we now look at coronary artery disease, and the major risk factors that cause or contribute to it. In addition to discussing the causes and effects of each risk factor on cardiovascular health, we note some ways to avoid or minimize them. While not all risk factors can be eliminated entirely, the questions and answers in this section can help you identify heart-healthy lifestyle habits.

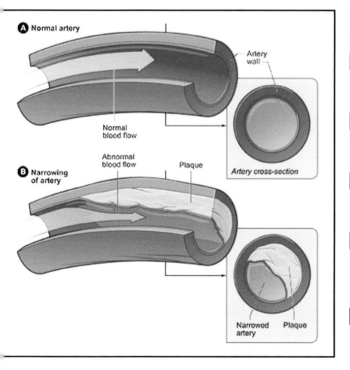

A Normal artery

Artery wall

Normal blood flow

Abnormal blood flow

Plaque

Artery cross-section

B Narrowing of artery

Narrowed artery

Plaque

Introduction to Heart Disease and Its Causes

6. What is heart disease?

Coronary heart disease (CHD) refers broadly to any disease or damage to the coronary arteries— the blood vessels that supply blood, oxygen, and nutrients to the heart—and is also called coronary artery disease.

DEFINITION

According to the Centers for Disease Control and Prevention (CDC), in 2008 over 405,000 people in the United States died from coronary heart disease.

NOTE

Most commonly, and for our purposes, CHD is a narrowing of the coronary arteries that results in diminished, or blocked, blood flow to the heart. Coronary heart disease

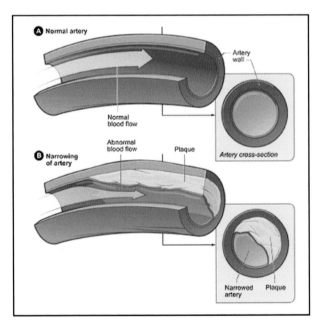

◄ FIGURE 4.1
Image of a clogged artery

SOURCE: http://www.nhlbi.nih.gov/health/health-topics/topics/cad/

is the leading cause of death in the United States for men and women.

 DEFINITION Atherosclerosis is the medical term for the build-up of fat, cholesterol, calcium, and other material found in the blood—together called **plaque**— on the inside lining of the arteries.

Coronary heart disease is most commonly caused by atherosclerosis.

This condition is also known as hardening of the arteries because it results in a loss of elasticity of the arteries. Atherosclerosis is one form of *arteriosclerosis*, which refers more generally to hardening of the arteries. Atherosclerosis is a form of arteriosclerosis that is specifically caused by the build-up of the plaque that underlies coronary heart disease.

Recent research suggests that dysfunction in the *endothelium*, the lining of the blood vessels, is a precursor to, and may be a predictor of, atherosclerosis. Endothelial cells are involved in coagulation and the adhesive properties of blood vessels, and it is thought that dysfunction of these cells may lead to, or contribute to, later development of atherosclerosis.

8. How does coronary heart disease affect the heart?

CHD can affect the coronary arteries and the heart in a number of ways.

1. First, the accumulation of plaque on the walls of the arteries can narrow them, which diminishes the amount of blood—and therefore oxygen and nutrients—available to the heart.

2. Second, plaque in the arteries can trigger an immune response, causing inflammation of the arteries and accumulation of white blood cells.

3. Finally, plaque may accumulate to the point that it either blocks the artery entirely, or plaque may break off or rupture, causing a clot that travels to a smaller artery and blocks the blood flow through that artery. If a coronary artery is blocked, the heart tissue that normally receives blood from that artery will be deprived of oxygen and nutrients, and can be significantly damaged, or die. This is a heart attack, or *myocardial infarction*.

Watch how a blood vessel narrows and becomes blocked.

http://footage.shutterstock.com/clip-1218184-stock-footage-atherosclerosis-cholesterol-plaque-forms-in-artery-ruptures-blood-clot-forms-and-artery-blocked.html

ON THE DVD

9. What are the risk factors associated with coronary heart disease?

There are a number of risk factors known to cause, or contribute to, coronary heart disease, and they will be discussed in following chapters. Risk factors include:

- High cholesterol, fats, and triglycerides in the blood
- High blood pressure (hypertension)
- Diabetes or pre-diabetes
- Obesity
- Smoking/use of oral tobacco products
- Lack of physical activity and exercise
- Excessive alcohol consumption
- Unhealthy diet
- Family history of heart disease
- Stress

According to the CDC, the chart below indicates the percentage of adults in the United States with coronary heart disease risk factors in 2005–2008.

NOTE

Some factors, such as high blood pressure and obesity, may run in families and create a genetic predisposition for that risk factor, and likewise, some people may be genetically predisposed to coronary heart disease generally. It is important to be aware if there is a history of heart disease in your family so that you can be vigilant in getting regular medical check-ups that include testing for heart disease. But even with a family history of heart disease, the risks of each of these contributing factors to heart disease can moderated to some extent—sometimes significantly—by lifestyle changes.

RISK FACTOR	%
Inactivity	53
Obesity	34
High Blood Pressure	32
Cigarette Smoking	21
High Cholesterol	15
Diabetes	11

Cholesterol, Triglycerides, and Fats as Risk Factors for Heart Disease

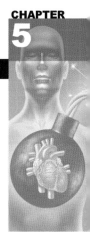

CHAPTER 5

10. What is cholesterol?

DEFINITION

Cholesterol is a waxy, lipid-based *sterol* (a combination of steroid and alcohol) that is naturally present in the body and serves a number of important functions.

Cholesterol is an essential component of cell membranes that cover the cells in our body. It is also important to the body's manufacture of bile, a substance stored in the gall

LDL cholesterol is known as "bad cholesterol" because it can permeate the walls of blood vessels and build up under them. LDL cholesterol is a main component of the plaque that can accumulate in the arteries and eventually narrow or block them. On the other hand, HDL cholesterol is known as "good cholesterol" because it helps fight the accumulation of harmful plaque, and it picks up excess cholesterol in the blood and carries it to the liver where it is broken down. Thus, LDL contributes to cardiovascular disease, while HDL serves to prevent it.

bladder that helps digest fats in food. Cholesterol aids in the absorption and metabolism of fat-soluble vitamins, such as vitamins A, D, E, and K. Roughly 70–75% of cholesterol is made in the body, and 25–30% comes from the food you eat.

Cholesterol is transported through the body by attaching to **lipoproteins**—proteins that carry lipids (very generally, certain fats and fat-based or fat-soluble substances). For our purposes, there are two main types of lipoproteins that carry cholesterol—**low-density lipoproteins (LDL)** and **high-density lipoproteins (HDL)**.

11. What is the healthy level of cholesterol?

A medical professional can perform a *lipid profile* on a blood sample to determine the levels of HDL, LDL, and total cholesterol, as well as the triglyceride level. Triglycerides are another form of fat, derived partially from food we eat, that can adversely affect cardiovascular health. Triglycerides are discussed in Questions 16–19.

Cholesterol levels are expressed as milligrams of cholesterol per volume of blood. In the United States, cholesterol is measured in mg/dL. (In Canada and most European countries, cholesterol levels are measured differently, in

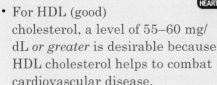

- For total cholesterol, a level of *less than* 200 mg/dL is desirable.
- For HDL (good) cholesterol, a level of 55–60 mg/dL *or greater* is desirable because HDL cholesterol helps to combat cardiovascular disease.
- For LDL (bad) cholesterol, a level of 100 mg/dL *or lower* is desirable because LDL cholesterol contributes to cardiovascular disease.

mmol/L.) A lipid profile will include at least three cholesterol measurements—total, HDL, and LDL cholesterol.

Because total cholesterol includes both good and bad types of cholesterol, it is best evaluated together with the individual HDL and LDL cholesterol levels. Medical authorities are divided on whether the LDL or HDL cholesterol level is more important. Some suggest that the LDL cholesterol level is more important because a high number indicates a higher risk of heart disease. Others take the view that the HDL cholesterol level is more important because HDL cholesterol helps cleanse the blood of bad cholesterol, and also protects the cardiovascular system from plaque build-up. Figure 5.1 shows cholesterol levels and

 Want to learn more about total cholesterol and LDL numbers? Visit:

http://www.nhlbi.nih.gov/health/public/heart/chol/wyntk.htm#numbers

▼ FIGURE 5.1
Cholesterol numbers and risk to heart health

TOTAL CHOLESTEROL	RISK CATEGORY
Less than 200	Desirable
200–239	Borderline high
240 and above	High

LDL CHOLESTEROL	LDL RISK CATEGORY
Less than 100	Optimal
100–129	Near optimal
130–159	Borderline high
160–189	High
190 and above	Very high

HDL	HDL RISK CATEGORY
60 or more	Desirable—helps to lower risk of heart disease
Less than 40	Major risk factor for heart disease

corresponding cardiovascular risk for the three cholesterol measurements.

Because a high HDL cholesterol level is beneficial to cardiovascular health and is included in your total cholesterol, another measure of your overall cholesterol profile is the ratio of total cholesterol to HDL cholesterol. For example, if your total cholesterol is 210 (slightly higher than the target level of 200) and your HDL cholesterol is 60 (very good), your ratio is 210/60, or 3.5:1, a very favorable ratio. The consensus among medical authorities is that:

- A ratio of 3.5 to 1 or lower (as in the above example) is optimal and helps to protect your heart;
- A ratio of 4 to 1 is satisfactory (e.g., 200 total/ 50 HDL); and
- A ratio of 5 to 1 or greater increases your risk of heart disease (e.g., 275 total/55 HDL).

In the example detailed above, a highly favorable HDL cholesterol level of 60 resulted in an optimal ratio even though total cholesterol of 210 was slightly higher than would normally be considered desirable.

12. What factors affect cholesterol levels?

There are a number of factors known to affect cholesterol levels:

- Lack of regular exercise
- Diet
- Being overweight
- Smoking
- Age and gender
- Family history
- Certain medical conditions and medications

13. How does regular exercise help to improve cholesterol levels?

Regular exercise is proven to have a number of beneficial effects on cardiovascular health, including both lowering LDL (bad) cholesterol and raising HDL (good) cholesterol. Researchers are not entirely certain how exercise specifically reduces bad cholesterol. There is some evidence that exercise stimulates the production of certain enzymes that help transport LDL cholesterol from the blood and blood vessel walls to the liver to be converted to bile or excreted. Some research also suggests that exercise may increase the size of cholesterol-carrying lipoproteins, reducing the possibility that they will enter blood vessels walls and contribute to the build-up of dangerous plaque.

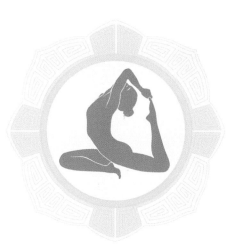

While some researchers believe that regular exercise helps raise the level of good cholesterol, the degree to which this occurs, and the physiology of how it works, is neither clear nor universally acknowledged in the medical community. Some research suggests that exercise helps to raise good cholesterol levels because exercise is associated with higher levels of certain lipoprotein-related enzymes, which may in turn be associated with higher HDL levels.

14. How does diet affect cholesterol levels?

Although only 25–30% of your cholesterol comes from food you eat, you can reduce your risk of cholesterol-related heart disease by avoiding foods that raise bad cholesterol and lower good cholesterol, and eating more foods that may boost good cholesterol. Diet can increase bad (LDL) cholesterol in two ways. First, only foods from animal sources contain cholesterol, and some are known to be high in LDL cholesterol such as:

- Egg yolks
- High fat dairy products such as whole milk, cheese, ice cream, and butter
- Fatty cuts of meat and poultry, particularly organs such as the liver
- Certain seafood such as shrimp, lobster, and shellfish (clams, oysters, and mussels)

Most people should limit cholesterol intake to less than 300 mg per day. If you have coronary heart disease or your LDL cholesterol level is 100 mg/dL or greater, limit your cholesterol intake to less than 200 milligrams a day. Cholesterol content is listed on most packaged food. For a comprehensive listing of the cholesterol content of packaged and prepared foods, see the **USDA National Nutrient Database for Standard Reference, Release 17** at:

http://nal.usda.gov/fnic/foodcomp/Data/SR17/wtrank/sr17w601.pdf

It is important to remember that many foods high in cholesterol, such as those noted above, also contain many nutrients that we need—such as protein, vitamins, minerals, and "good" fats. Unless you have been advised by your medical professional to minimize all higher cholesterol foods, occasional consumption of modest portions of these foods may be part of a balanced diet.

Reducing consumption of these types of foods will reduce adding bad cholesterol to your body. On the other hand, foods from plant sources—such as fruits, nuts, vegetables, and legumes—do not contain cholesterol but they do have many valuable nutrients.

Second, in addition to the consumption of foods with high cholesterol content, a diet that is high in certain kinds of fat (the "bad fats") can also increase the level of LDL cholesterol. The main fats that contribute to higher LDL cholesterol levels are **saturated fat** and **trans fat**. These are discussed in more detail in the next question. So eat fewer high-LDL foods, more low-LDL foods, and fewer "bad fat" foods.

In addition to reducing your cardiovascular risk by avoiding foods with high LDL cholesterol and bad fats, there is some evidence, not yet definitively proven, that foods rich in unsaturated fats may help raise HDL (good) cholesterol and therefore contribute to cardiovascular health. These foods are listed in Question 15.

 How smart are you when it comes to cholesterol? Take the American Heart Association's Cholesterol Quiz!

http://www.heart.org/HEARTORG/
Conditions/Cholesterol/AboutCholesterol/
Cholesterol-IQ-Quiz_UCM_305563_
Article.jsp

15. I'm confused about fats—what do I need to know?

There are several different kinds of fat in food—some bad, some good—but with basic information and dietary tips, you can dramatically improve the "fat profile" of your diet and reduce this risk to heart health. Here are the main things to know about fat in foods and cardiovascular health.

Saturated fat is generally considered one of the "bad" fats because the current consensus among health professionals is that it raises the risk of cardiovascular disease. Although there is a lack of strong definitive evidence of a direct link between saturated fat and heart disease, saturated fat is thought to contribute to the build-up of plaque in the arteries, and may also contribute to higher LDL (bad) cholesterol levels. Most saturated fat comes from animal food sources, but there are also plant food sources of saturated fat. Examples of each include:

- Fattier cuts of beef, lamb, veal, and poultry
- Coconut oil and palm oil

Foods high in saturated fat are often the same foods that are high in LDL cholesterol. Even without proof of a direct correlation between saturated fat intake and cardiovascular risk, most health professionals—including the American Heart Association—recommend limiting, or at least moderating, the consumption of foods with high saturated fat content.

Trans fat (short for "trans fatty acids") is the other main type of bad fat and refers to vegetable oils that have undergone a chemical process called "partial hydrogenation." They are most commonly used in commercial cooking and baking, and in making margarine. Too much trans fat poses a significant threat to heart health because it can raise your LDL (bad) cholesterol levels and lower your HDL (good) cholesterol levels. Trans fats have typically been present in baked goods such as cookies, crackers, muffins, pastries, and pizza dough, and in deep-fried food like french fries. Because of the clear link between trans fat in the diet and cardiovascular disease, companies are starting to use healthier alternatives in their food products—especially since the United States Food and Drug Administration began requiring packaged food sold in stores to specifically list trans fat content on the label.

Unsaturated fat (including monounsaturated fat and polyunsaturated fat) is considered a healthier type of fat than saturated fat. Some studies suggest that diets high in unsaturated fat may help lower LDL (bad) cholesterol levels and therefore lower the risk of heart disease. Additionally, unsaturated fat may help control blood sugar and insulin levels, reducing the risk of developing Type 2 diabetes, or helping moderate its effects in people who already have it. Foods high in unsaturated fat include:

- Vegetable oils, such as olive, canola, peanut, and corn oils
- Avocados and olives
- Nuts, such as almonds, cashews, walnuts, and hazelnuts
- Seeds, such as pumpkin seeds and sesame seeds
- Fattier fish, such as salmon, trout, and halibut

The American Heart Association recommends that children and adults:

HEART HEALTH

- Limit total fat intake to less than 25–35% of your total calories each day (the U.S. Food and Drug Administration recommends no greater than 30%);
- Limit saturated fat intake to less than 7% of total daily calories;
- Limit *trans* fat intake to less than 1% of total daily calories; and
- The remaining fat should come from sources of monounsaturated and polyunsaturated fats such as nuts, seeds, fish, and vegetable oils.

16. What are triglycerides?

Triglycerides are a specific type of lipid (fat) that are present in certain types of food, and are also manufactured by the body from fat and carbohydrates in our diet. Their main function is to store and transport the substances that the body converts to energy when the body needs it. When the body does not use dietary fat and carbohydrates for energy after we eat, the excess is metabolized into triglycerides and stored in the liver and fat cells. When your body needs energy that is not immediately supplied by food intake, specific hormones release and break down the triglycerides into usable forms for metabolic functions that call for the stored energy.

17. Why are triglycerides a risk factor for heart disease?

While triglycerides serve an important function, like cholesterol, too high a level presents a significant risk to cardiovascular health, particularly the accumulation of plaque in the arteries. However, it is not entirely clear how a high triglyceride level directly contributes to cardiovascular risk. Research indicates that high triglyceride levels have a high correlation to other cardiovascular risks, such as high cholesterol, obesity, high blood sugar (diabetes), and high blood pressure.

18. How are triglycerides measured, and what is a healthy level?

Triglycerides are typically measured with cholesterol as part of a lipid profile through a blood test. Like cholesterol, in the United States triglyceride levels are expressed in milligrams per volume of blood (mg/dL). The chart below sets forth commonly accepted triglyceride guidelines.

Less than 100 mg/dL	optimal (may improve heart health)
Less than 150 mg/dL	normal
150–199 mg/dL	borderline high
200–499 mg/dL	high

19. How can I work toward a healthy triglyceride level?

Also like cholesterol, triglycerides are believed to contribute to the build-up of plaque in the arteries, including the coronary arteries, and the ways to work toward healthy levels are similar: regular moderate exercise, reducing the intake of foods high in cholesterol, saturated fats, and trans fats, and reducing alcohol consumption. Alcohol consumption in particular has a high correlation to triglyceride accumulation. Finally, diets high in carbohydrates (sugars) stimulate insulin production, and this has been shown to increase triglyceride levels. When lifestyle changes are not enough to reduce blood triglycerides to healthy levels, your doctor may prescribe medication to further reduce triglyceride levels. Medications commonly used to control triglyceride levels are the same ones used to control high cholesterol, such as statins, as well as an omega-3 based drug called Lovaza.

20. What are omega-3 fatty acids?

Omega-3 fatty acids are a type of polyunsaturated fat that have been shown to be particularly effective in reducing the risk of heart disease. Omega-3 fatty acids are considered *essential fatty acids* because they are essential to our health, but they are not produced in the body so they must be obtained from our food. Research has shown that populations of people whose diet consists of high amounts of oily fish—salmon, tuna, mackerel, herring, and trout—have very low rates of heart disease. Health professionals recommend eating high omega-3 foods twice a week. Doctors and nutritionists may recommend that people who have heart disease, or are at a high risk of getting heart disease, take fish oil or other omega-3 supplements.

Blood Pressure as a Risk Factor for Heart Disease

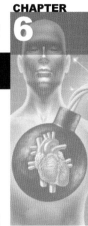

21. What is blood pressure and why do I need to know about it?

DEFINITION

Blood pressure is the force, or pressure, of blood pushing against the walls of the arteries as the heart pumps blood through the body.

It is very important to understand and monitor your blood pressure, and to maintain it at a proper level. If it is too high—called high blood pressure or *hypertension*—you are at a much higher risk of coronary heart disease. High blood pressure is a common medical condition that affects 1 in 4 American adults. It is often referred to as "the silent killer" because many people who suffer from high blood pressure

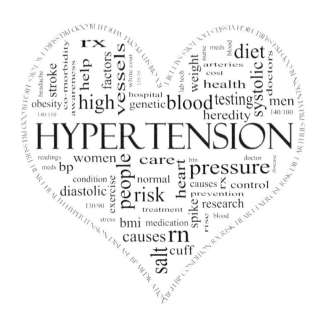

have no obvious symptoms. Therefore, a person can have high blood pressure for years without knowing it—while the adverse affects can accumulate in various parts of the body—so it is important to monitor your blood pressure periodically.

22. How is blood pressure measured?

There are two components to a blood pressure measurement. One component is the pressure in the arteries when the heart contracts and pumps blood, pushing it against the walls of the arteries. This is called the *systolic pressure*. The other component is the pressure in the arteries between heartbeats when the heart is at rest. This is called the *diastolic pressure*. Medical professionals usually measure blood pressure using a *sphygmomanometer*, which is a pressure gauge graduated in millimeters of mercury, and a stethoscope. An inflatable cuff is placed around the upper arm, inflated to compress an artery, and then slowly deflated while the stethoscope is used to listen to the blood flow through the artery to determine when the heart beats, and when it is at rest. At these two points, the systolic and diastolic pressures are observed on the pressure gauge. Whatever type of measuring instrument is used, systolic and diastolic pressures are expressed in millimeters of mercury.

23. What do blood pressure numbers mean?

Systolic and diastolic blood pressures are expressed in millimeters of mercury, with the systolic pressure indicated first. The commonly accepted normal blood pressure in an adult at rest is 120/80. This refers to a systolic pressure of 120 and a diastolic pressure of 80. Accounting for slight variation among healthy adults:

- The normal range systolic blood pressure is 120–130, and
- The normal range for diastolic pressure is 72–84.

Blood pressure consistently higher than those ranges—absent other factors—is indicative of high blood pressure, or hypertension, and carries the risk of negative health effects.

The degree to which blood pressure exceeds these norms determines the severity—and accompanying risks—of high blood pressure. The categories of blood pressure in adults are:

- Normal (120/80)
- Pre-hypertension (120–140/80–90)
- High Blood Pressure Stage 1 (140–160/90–100)
- High Blood Pressure Stage 2 (over 160/over 100)

Blood pressure typically rises with age, and this may be taken into account when assessing whether a person's blood pressure is too high. The following chart shows normal blood pressures for men and women at various ages.

Blood Pressure for Men and Women at Ages 10–74

Age in Years	SYSTOLIC PRESSURE		DIASTOLIC PRESSURE	
	Men	Women	Men	Women
10	102	102	68	70
11	104	104	70	71
12	106	106	70	72
13	108	108	72	74
14	110	110	72	74
15	112	112	74	76
16	118	116	74	72
17	120	116	74	72
18	120	116	74	72
19	122	116	76	72
20–24	124	116	76	72
25–29	126	118	78	74
30–34	126	120	78	76
35–39	128	124	80	78
40–44	130	128	82	80
45–49	130	132	82	82
50–54	136	138	82	84
55–59	138	140	84	84

	SYSTOLIC PRESSURE		DIASTOLIC PRESSURE	
Age in Years	Men	Women	Men	Women
60–64	142	144	86	86
65–69	144	154	84	86
70–74	146	160	82	86

24. Why does high blood pressure (hypertension) increase the risk of heart disease?

High blood pressure increases the risk of cardiovascular and heart disease in a number of related ways. High blood pressure means that the flow of blood is putting extra force against the lining of the arteries. The stress of this extra force can damage the arteries, and damaged arteries are more susceptible to the accumulation of plaque, which narrows them. This creates a dangerous cycle, because as the arteries begin to narrow, blood has to flow against greater resistance, and blood pressure may rise still further—resulting in more arterial damage and more accumulation of plaque.

In addition to being a high risk factor for heart disease, high blood pressure also increases the risks of other health problems, including kidney disease, stroke (the blockage of blood flow through an artery in the brain), aneurysm (a rupture of an artery), and eye damage.

25. What causes high blood pressure?

Your doctor may not be able to identify a specific cause for high blood pressure. High blood pressure that cannot be attributed to a specific cause is called *essential* or *primary hypertension*, and over 90% of people with high blood pressure fall into this category. While the specific cause of essential hypertension may not be clear, there are a number of factors known to cause or contribute to it. These factors include:

- Family history of high blood pressure (genetics)
- Obesity

- Lack of regular exercise
- Smoking
- Advanced age
- High caffeine intake in the form of coffee or tea
- Diet high in fats and oils (especially saturated fats)
- High cholesterol levels
- High salt (sodium) intake
- Type 2 diabetes
- Excessive alcohol intake
- Stress

In addition, certain segments of the population are at greater risk of high blood pressure, such as pregnant women, women taking birth control pills, and African-Americans.

High blood pressure that can be attributed to a specific cause is called *secondary hypertension*, and is usually caused by other medical conditions or medications. Medical conditions that can cause secondary hypertension include diabetes, kidney disease, endocrine disorders, pregnancy, sleep apnea, or a birth defect that causes a narrowing of the aorta. Medications that can cause secondary hypertension include nonsteroidal anti-inflammatory drugs (NSAIDs) such as ibuprofen (like Advil or Motrin) and naproxen (Aleve), corticosteroids, and oral contraceptives. Cold remedy decongestants that contain pseudoephedrine can worsen high blood pressure in people who already have it. Because secondary hypertension is treated as part of the treatment of the underlying cause, or by addressing any other medication that may be causing it, we will limit our discussion to primary hypertension.

26. How can high blood pressured be controlled and treated?

People who have been diagnosed with high blood pressure should work closely with a medical professional to determine an appropriate treatment regimen. In some cases, blood pressure may be returned to and maintained at healthy levels through lifestyle changes. Referring back to the list of causes and contributing factors to high blood pressure in Question 25:

- If you are overweight, talk to a medical professional about healthy weight loss
- If your doctor confirms that it is safe for you to do so, get regular exercise
- Stop using tobacco products
- Reduce your caffeine intake
- Reduce the amount of saturated and other harmful types of fat in your diet
- Discuss cholesterol reduction with your doctor
- Reduce your sodium intake
- Discuss your alcohol consumption with your doctor
- Explore ways to reduce stress

In addition to lifestyle changes that have been shown to reduce high blood pressure, there are several types of drugs used to treat high blood pressure, including:

- Angiotensin-converting enzyme (ACE) inhibitors
- Angiotensin II receptor blockers (ARBs)
- Diuretics
- Beta-blockers
- Calcium channel blockers
- Alpha blockers
- Alpha 2 receptor agonists
- Renin inhibitors

Each type of drug works somewhat differently, and is prescribed to patients based on their individual circumstances as well as other health issues, potential side effects, and other medications. Because high blood pressure is a significant risk factor for heart and other cardiovascular disease—as well as other serious health problems—it must be monitored regularly and kept under control.

Diabetes as a Risk Factor for Heart Disease

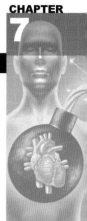

CHAPTER 7

27. What is diabetes?

Diabetes is a medical condition in which the body's blood sugar levels are too high. This is a result of the body's inability to make enough of a hormone called insulin, or because the cells in the body do not properly use the insulin that the body does produce. Insulin is what helps the body metabolize sugar, so if you don't make enough insulin, or don't use what you have, there will be too much sugar in the blood. There are three types of diabetes: Type 1 (formerly known as juvenile diabetes), in which the body does not make insulin; Type 2, in which the body does not make enough insulin or the body's cells do not use available insulin; and gestational diabetes, in which pregnant women develop diabetes. While some research suggests that gestational diabetes may be a precursor for future Type 2 diabetes, many women with gestational diabetes never develop Type 2 diabetes after pregnancy.

NOTE

In addition to increasing the risk of heart disease, diabetes increases the risk of stroke, kidney disease, eye disease, and a number of conditions related to impaired circulation.

28. Why is diabetes such a high risk factor for heart disease?

Type 1 and Type 2 diabetes is one of the most significant risk factors for coronary heart disease for two reasons. First, the high blood sugar levels resulting from diabetes increase the risk of cardiovascular disease because uncontrolled sugar levels can damage the lining of blood vessels. Second, diabetes substantially increases the frequency and adverse effects of several other risk factors for cardiovascular disease. According to the American Heart Association, there is a strong correlation between diabetes and a number of other heart disease risk factors, including high blood pressure, high cholesterol, and obesity. In addition, the presence of diabetes increases the risk of cardiovascular disease in people who smoke to an even greater degree than the risk for non-diabetic smokers. It is therefore critically important that people with diabetes work to both maintain normal and stable blood sugar levels, and to try to minimize the effects of other heart disease risk factors.

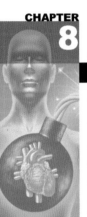

Obesity as a Risk Factor for Heart Disease

CHAPTER 8

29. How is "obesity" defined and measured?

The term "obesity" has been variously described as having too much body fat for your body size, or too much body fat as a proportion of your body weight, or being significantly over your healthy body weight due to too much fat. The key criterion is weight that is attributable to fat. In contrast, for example, a trained athlete may be over a generally accepted body weight due to significant muscle development and not be susceptible to weight-related health risks.

The body will tend to gain unhealthy weight when you consume more calories—the measure of energy content in foods—than your body needs. Fat contains the highest amount of calories of the food we eat—about 9 calories per gram. In contrast, carbohydrates and protein each contain about 4 calories per gram. Alcohol—often overlooked as a contributor to body weight—contains about 7 calories per gram. When the body is given more calories than it needs for metabolic activity and the growth and maintenance of tissue, it has a tendency to store the excess as fat.

30. What is Body Mass Index (BMI)?

The most common measure of weight health is the Body Mass Index (BMI), which factors in your height and body weight to determine if you are carrying a healthy proportion of body fat. Adult men and women can calculate their BMI as follows:

1. Multiply your weight (in pounds) by 703

2. Divide that number by your height (in inches)

3. Divide that number by your height again

For example, a woman who is 5'6" (66 inches) and weighs 170 pounds would have a BMI of [(703 x 170) ÷ 66] ÷ 66 = 27.4. The chart below sets forth the ranges of BMI and corresponding category of weight health.

BMI	CATEGORY
Below 18.5	Underweight
18.5–24.9	Healthy
25.0–29.9	Overweight
30.0–39.9	Obese
40 and above	Morbidly obese

So in the example above, the woman with a BMI of 27.4 would be considered overweight. While BMI is a generally accepted indicator of unhealthy weight, note that a BMI of 30—the threshold for obesity—is only 20% above the healthy range. According to the American Heart Association, between 60% and 70% of American adults have a BMI in the overweight or obese category. For many people who fall into these categories, lifestyle changes help get them to a healthier BMI, and therefore reduce the health risk of being overweight.

 An excellent BMI calculator is located online at:

http://www.crestor.com/c/your-arteries/tools-resources/bmi-calculator.aspx

BMI is calculated the same way for men and women regardless of age and the BMI/risk categories are also the same. However, men and women typically have different proportions of body fat, and older adults tend to have more body fat than younger ones, so you should discuss your specific situation with your doctor.

31. Is BMI calculated and interpreted the same way for children?

BMI is calculated the same way for children and teenagers as it is for adults. However, because the amount of body fat of children and teenagers changes with age and by sex, there are separate age- and sex-specific charts that take these differences into consideration.

For an assessment of BMI and BMI category for children and teens ages 2–19, go to:

TOOLS

http://apps.nccd.cdc.gov/dnpabmi/

32. Does BMI really measure body fat, or are there other methods?

It is important to keep in mind that BMI is not a direct measure of body fat, but rather a measure of body weight per a given height. Body weight also includes bone and muscle, which are both denser than fat, so a person with more bone or muscle mass will often have a BMI in the Overweight category but not have an unhealthy body fat content. The BMI is a screening tool for unhealthy weight, but it is not a direct measuring or diagnostic tool. There are a number of ways to measure body fat, from one as simple as measuring skin fold thickness with calipers, to underwater weighing and biometrical impedance (seeing how fast a weak electric current travels through you), to more elaborate and expensive techniques such as dual-energy X-ray absorptiometry.

33. What causes obesity?

There are several widely known causes for obesity. The tendency to be overweight often runs in families. And some people have a greater metabolic tendency to gain and retain weight. Aside from a genetic or metabolic predisposition toward obesity, lifestyle habits are the biggest causes of obesity, including eating too much food in general, consuming too much high fat foods, high alcohol intake, and lack of regular exercise—each of which contributes to consuming more calories than your body can use. There are a number of other causes of weight gain, such as taking certain medications and certain medical conditions. It is important to discuss concerns about weight gain and healthy weight loss with your medical professional.

34. Why is obesity a high risk factor for heart disease?

First, obesity can cause changes in the structure and function of the heart, even for an otherwise healthy person with no other risk factors and no atherosclerosis. Carrying too much unhealthy weight requires the heart to work harder to pump blood through the extra body mass, and this added stress can expand and stretch the heart muscle causing it to get thicker, and lose its normal elasticity and its capacity to contract. Over time, the heart may start to lose its ability to fully expand and contract as it beats, resulting in impaired circulation of oxygen-rich blood through the body, especially during activity or exercise. This condition is called *heart failure*. Further, when the heart is unable to efficiently move blood through the body, fluids may build up in the lungs, other organs, and arms and legs—a condition called *congestive heart failure*.

In addition to the direct health risks it poses to the heart, obesity is a major risk factor for heart disease for several other reasons, including:

- It raises blood pressure
- It raises bad cholesterol and lowers good cholesterol
- It raises the risk of diabetes

35. How can obesity be controlled?

Assuming your doctor has determined that there is no specific medical condition causing obesity, the way to reduce unhealthy weight is to take in fewer calories and burn more—simply put, eat less, eat fewer high fat foods, and get more exercise. If you reduce your calorie intake, and get regular, moderate exercise, your body will start to use stored fat for energy and this will lead to a gradual loss of unhealthy weight. Before starting an exercise regimen, consult with your doctor to confirm that it is safe to do so, and how to safely build up the type, frequency, and intensity of exercise. Because the heart of an overweight body is already working extra hard, and may already be at risk of atherosclerosis, anyone starting out to lose weight through exercise must do so under their doctor's direction.

Nutritionists recommend that adult men consume an average of 2000–2500 calories per day, and women, 1800–2300 calories per day. Individual needs will vary by body size and level of activity.

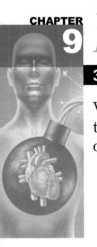

To look up the nutritional content of thousands of foods, including fat content, visit the United States Department of Agriculture's Nutrient Database at:

http://ndb.nal.usda.gov/

If you plan to lose unhealthy weight through a combination of diet and exercise, here's the formula to do the numbers: 3500 calories from food intake = one pound of fat. This means that to lose one pound of excess body fat, you need to burn 3500 more calories than you take in.

Smoking and Other Tobacco Products as Risk Factors for Heart Disease

CHAPTER 9

36. How does smoking increase the risk of heart disease?

Virtually everyone knows that smoking is very dangerous to your health. Here are the many reasons why smoking is one of the greatest risk factors specifically for heart disease:

- Smoking increases LDL (bad) cholesterol.
- Smoking increases the build-up of plaque in the arteries.
- Smoking increases clotting.
- Smoking lowers HDL (good) cholesterol.
- Smoking damages the lining of blood vessels (endothelium).

- Smoking temporarily increases blood pressure.
- Smoking can cause spasms in the coronary arteries.

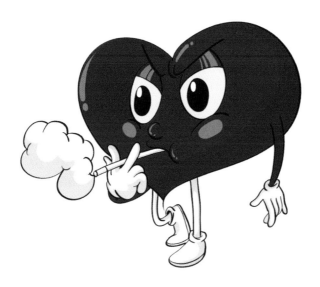

37. Can the harmful health effects of smoking be reversed if you stop?

For the most part, yes—anyone who quits smoking will have both short-term and long-term health benefits. The degree to which quitting smoking can reverse the accumulated damage will depend on things like how long you smoked, how much you smoked, what age you started smoking, and what age you stop. But regardless of these variables, quitting smoking will result in greatly improved health.

Quitting smoking will stop further damage to your cardiovascular system as well as the spikes in blood pressure that nicotine causes. Over the long term, quitting smoking will dramatically reduce the damage to the cardiovascular system caused by the effects of smoking set forth in Question 36. After many years of not smoking, the risk of developing heart disease will decrease almost to the same level as a person who never smoked, independent of the presence of the other risk factors for heart disease. We discuss quitting smoking in detail in Chapter 17.

38. Does "smokeless" tobacco also present a risk for cardiovascular disease?

By smokeless tobacco, we mean products such as chewing tobacco and snuff that are used in the mouth. Research has not found that smokeless tobacco presents all of the same risks to cardiovascular health as smoking. However, because it contains high amounts of nicotine, smokeless tobacco raises blood pressure and heart rate, and is therefore unhealthy for the heart and cardiovascular system. In addition, smokeless tobacco presents many other serious risks, such as oral cancers, gum disease, tooth decay, and addiction. Health professionals do not consider smokeless tobacco to be a safe alternative form of tobacco use to smoking.

Lack of Physical Activity and Exercise as a Risk Factor for Heart Disease

CHAPTER 10

39. Why is lack of physical activity a risk factor for heart disease?

We have touched briefly in prior questions on the benefits of regular exercise for cardiovascular heath. But unlike other risk factors, lack of exercise does not by itself *cause* heart disease. Rather, a lack of exercise represents the absence of one of the very important and effective components of good cardiovascular health because exercise can help to lessen the harmful effects of several other significant risk factors.

And the doctor says, "When you get up in the morning, take an aspirin. . . for a brisk walk, then to the gym, then take it for a bike ride. . ."

HEART HEALTH

Exercise is important to cardiovascular health because:

1. The heart is a muscle, and making it work during regular exercise serves to strengthen it just like when you regularly work other muscles in the body. A stronger heart can pump more blood with less work—to keep up with added demands of physical exertion, as well to work less strenuously when the body is at rest.

2. Exercise improves the function of the endothelia, the lining of the blood vessels through which the transfer of oxygen and nutrients takes place.

3. Exercise improves circulation and can help reduce the symptoms of congestive heart failure.

In addition to the direct benefits to the cardiovascular system, regular exercise also helps fight other risk factors because it:

- Lowers blood pressure
- Lowers LDL (bad) cholesterol
- Raises HDL (good) cholesterol
- Lowers trigycerides
- Lowers body fat (when combined with a healthy diet)

41. What are the types of exercise that are best for cardiovascular health?

Most exercise falls into one of two categories—**aerobic** and **anaerobic**—and some forms of exercise involve both. They differ in the intensity and duration of the activity, involve different metabolic processes for the production of the energy required, and have different benefits to health.

Aerobic exercise—literally meaning "with oxygen"—is exercise of lower physical intensity and longer duration than anaerobic exercise. Aerobic exercise uses oxygen to burn fat for the energy required, and can be performed for extended periods of time as long as the cardiovascular system can supply enough oxygen-rich blood to the muscles involved. Common examples include walking briskly, jogging, aerobic dance, swimming, using a stair machine or elliptical trainer, or bicycling.

On the other hand, **anaerobic exercise**—meaning "without oxygen"—is exercise of high physical intensity and much shorter duration. Anaerobic exercise requires a greater amount of short-term energy than the body can produce by using oxygen to burn fat, and instead relies on a process that breaks down a compound that is stored in the muscle to release glucose (sugar) as the energy source. This energy-producing process does not rely on oxygen (and is therefore anaerobic), but can only be carried out for very short periods. Common examples include strength training/weight lifting and sprinting. While anaerobic exercise provides a number of health benefits, such as increased strength, increased muscle mass, and fat reduction because of a higher metabolic rate at rest, aerobic exercise provides greater benefits to cardiovascular health.

42. How does aerobic exercise support cardiovascular health?

Regular aerobic exercise can:

- Lower your blood pressure. Exercise strengthens the heart muscle, enabling it to pump more blood with less effort. More efficient pumping decreases the stress—or pressure—on the artery walls. It can take one to three months to achieve this benefit, but studies have shown that for some people regular exercise can lower blood pressure as effectively as medication.

- Improve cholesterol levels. While research in this area is not firmly conclusive, there is substantial evidence that regular exercise boosts HDL (good) cholesterol levels, or at least prevents it from decreasing. To realize this benefit, the exercise needs to be more intense and more frequent than that required for other health benefits. Likewise, while studies have found a strong correlation between cardiovascular fitness and lower LDL (bad) cholesterol levels, the biochemical mechanism for the connection is unclear. However, most authorities on cardiovascular health agree that for many people, regular aerobic exercise will improve their cholesterol profile, and the more frequent and intense the exercise, the greater the effect.

- Lower triglyceride levels. Research in this area is clear—regular aerobic exercise can dramatically lower triglyceride levels as much as 25%. And unlike the high frequency and intensity required to achieve higher HDL cholesterol levels, improved triglyceride levels are observed with regular, but moderate exercise—for example, walking 12 miles per week.

- Lower body fat. Remember that, by definition, aerobic exercise means that the body is using oxygen to convert fat to energy. So the more energy you expend, the more fat you'll burn. While this often translates to weight loss, people who combine aerobic exercise with muscle building exercise may not experience weight loss—but they will still be lowering body fat.

43. How much exercise do I need to improve my heart and cardiovascular health?

In 2006, the United States Department of Health and Human Services, in its Physical Activity Guidelines for Americans, indicated that adults gain substantial health benefits from 2 ½ hours of moderate intensity aerobic physical activity, or 1 ¼ hours of vigorous physical activity per week. Examples of moderate intensity activity include:

- Walking briskly
- Water aerobics
- Ballroom dancing
- Gardening

Vigorous aerobic activities include:

- Racewalking
- Jogging or running

- Swimming laps
- Hiking uphill or with a heavy backpack

Not surprisingly, the more aerobic exercise you get, the greater the health benefits. You'll know when you can increase your amount of exercise when what you're doing becomes easier for you. More exercise can mean any combination of:

- Greater frequency, such as 5 times a week instead of 4,

- Greater intensity exercise, such as progressing from moderate to vigorous, or

- More time at each exercise or activity session, such as increasing from 30 to 45 minutes per session.

Including anaerobic exercise in your routine, such as weight and strength training, provides additional health benefits beyond what aerobic exercise alone typically offers. Regular anaerobic exercise can increase your overall metabolic rate, which burns calories and helps manage weight, helps build and maintain lean muscle tissue, and increases bone density and strength.

NOTE

While there is a point at which you're getting as much cardiovascular benefit as exercise can offer and more exercise will not offer more benefit, very few people reach that point.

CASE STUDY

While medical research may not be able to definitively explain each of the precise reasons *why* exercise helps combat several risk factors for heart disease, there is no debate that it does. See how starting even a modest routine of regular aerobic exercise improved the health profile of someone with common heart disease risk factors.

Mary is a 70 year-old woman with the following risk factors for heart disease:

- Body weight of 161 pounds with 40% body fat
- High systolic blood pressure (145/70) at rest

- Total cholesterol over 200 (undesirable) for which she was already taking a statin to help reduce it
- Borderline high LDL (bad) cholesterol of 145 mg/dl
- Total cholesterol/HDL cholesterol ratio of 4.9 (borderline increased risk of heart disease)
- Virtually no exercise other than errands and housework

Upon medical advice, Mary regularly participated in a supervised 12-week aerobic exercise program that consisted of 30 minutes of moderate intensity aerobic exercise 3 times per week. Mary chose a combination of brisk walking on a treadmill and pedaling a stationary bicycle.

At the end of the 12 weeks, Mary's risk factors were re-evaluated and showed the following:
- Body fat reduced from 40% to 37%
- Systolic blood pressure dropped from an unhealthy 145 to a very healthy 114 at rest
- Total cholesterol was reduced from over 200 mg/dl to 180 mg/dl (desirable)
- LDL cholesterol dropped from 145 (borderline high) to 115 (near optimal)
- Total cholesterol/HDL cholesterol ratio dropped from 4.9 to 4.1 (just slightly above the satisfactory threshold of 4.0)

Mary's medical team attributed each of these improvements in Mary's heart health profile to the addition of regular exercise to her weekly routine.

Adapted from the American Diabetes Association Clinical Diabetes Journal

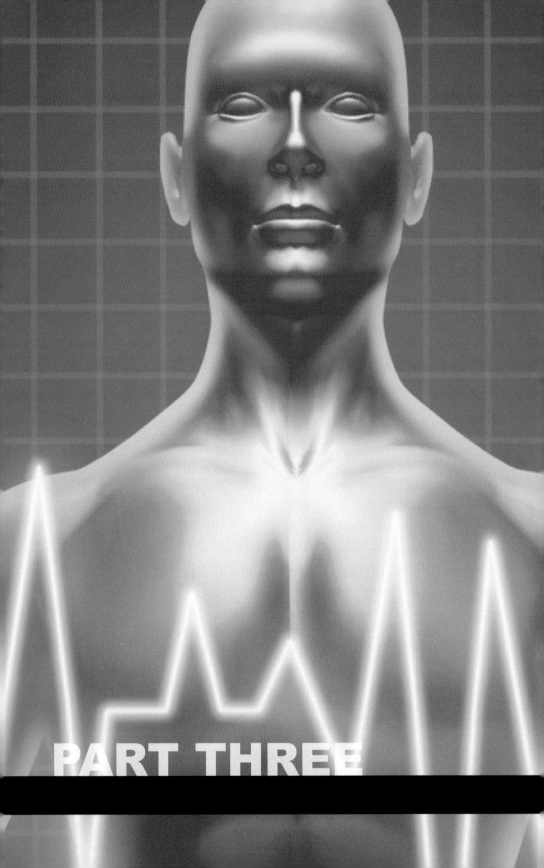

PART THREE

Symptoms and Diagnosis of Heart Disease and Treatment of a Heart Attack

In Part Three, we will look at physical symptoms and warning signs that may signal heart disease, and diagnostic tools used by medical professionals to determine the presence and severity of heart and coronary artery disease. We will then explain the symptoms, diagnosis, and emergency treatment of a heart attack.

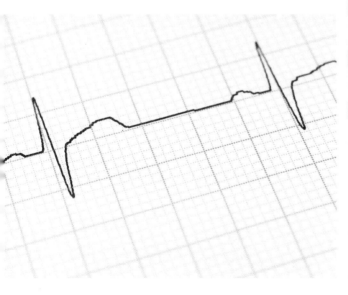

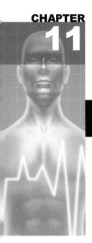

11 *Symptoms of Heart Disease*

44. What are the signs or symptoms of coronary heart disease?

There are a number of signs and symptoms of heart disease, including:

- Chest discomfort or pain (called *angina*)
- Shortness of breath for unexplained reasons
- Irregular heart rate, such as palpitations or the feeling that your heart is "racing"
- Dizziness or feeling weak
- Nausea
- Unexplained sweating
- Constant or frequent fatigue

According to the National Institutes of Health, 6 million American women have coronary heart disease. For more information, see CBS 19's Women's Heart Attack Symptoms at: http://www.youtube.com/watch?v=SPe8y4OeXQQ&feature=related

PRACTICAL TIP

45. What is angina?

Angina, or *angina pectoris*, refers to discomfort or pain in the chest, and in the absence of specific pain, may feel like pressure, heaviness, burning, aching, fullness, tightness, or squeezing in the chest. Angina is often caused by a narrowing of coronary arteries due to plaque, which is why it is often a symptom of heart disease. When the flow of oxygen and nutrients to the heart is impaired due to a narrowing or blockage in a coronary artery, the heart must use anaerobic sources of energy—those not oxygen dependent—to keep pumping blood. A by-product of anaerobic energy is lactic acid, and when lactic acid

According to the National Heart, Blood, and Lung Institute, experts believe that almost 7 million people in the United States suffer from angina, with equal numbers among men and women.

NOTE

builds up in any muscle—including the heart—that build up can cause pain or discomfort.

46. Are there different kinds of angina?

Yes, and it is important to understand the differences. Only a doctor can identify the type and source of angina that someone may be experiencing and prescribe an appropriate treatment.

Stable angina is the most common form of angina, and is characterized by a predictable pattern of chest pain most often brought on by physical or emotional stress. It generally subsides with rest, and may also be treated with medication. While stable angina is not usually a symptom of a heart attack, it increases the possibility of a heart attack in the future and people with this condition must be aware of its patterns and seek immediate medical attention if it worsens and does not respond as usual to rest and prescribed medication. Stable angina can be present even in the absence of cardiovascular disease; for example, people with certain heart valve problems or who have infections of the lung or lining of the heart may also experience stable angina.

Unstable angina is more dangerous than stable angina, and may signal an impending heart attack. Unstable angina:

- Does not follow a predictable pattern,
- May arise without physical or emotional stress,
- May have more intense pain or discomfort, and
- May not subside with rest or medication.

If you have not previously experienced angina, or if you have had stable angina but have an episode that is different from or worse than before and does not respond to usual treatment, seek immediate medical attention.

Variant (or *Prinzmetal's*) *angina* is a rare form of angina that occurs when there is a spasm in the coronary artery, causing the artery to temporarily narrow. It typically occurs when a person is sleeping or at rest, and may occur when someone is exposed to cold temperatures. Variant angina can be treated with medication.

47. Do men and women experience the same angina symptoms?

Some research shows that women are more likely to experience sharp pain rather than the less specific symptoms of pressure, heaviness, or a squeezing sensation in the chest. According to the Mayo Clinic, it may feel more like a stabbing or pulsating sensation. However, women are also more likely to feel discomfort in areas other than the chest, such as the neck, jaw, throat, or back, and may also experience abdominal discomfort and nausea more than men.

48. How is angina treated?

Angina is typically treated with a combination of lifestyle changes, medication, and surgical procedures—each depending on the type and severity of the angina as diagnosed by your doctor.

- Because angina is most often associated with coronary artery disease, the lifestyle changes recommended to alleviate angina are many of the same ones previously discussed to prevent or reduce the risks for cardiovascular disease generally (see Chapters 4–10):
  - Stop smoking
  - Avoid large meals and reduce the consumption of foods high in bad fats and cholesterol
  - Get regular, moderate aerobic exercise
  - Reduce unhealthy weight
  - Limit alcohol consumption
  - Avoid stress
  - Control your blood pressure

- If you have diabetes, control your blood sugar and insulin levels

There are different classes of medications prescribed to prevent and treat angina, and while they work differently and may also be prescribed for other conditions, they share some similar effects. Following are three of the most common:

- The most commonly prescribed medications are *nitrates*, which relax and widen blood vessels to allow blood to flow more easily through them with less work from the heart. Nitroglycerin is a nitrate used to relieve or prevent an angina attack. It is placed under the tongue or between cheek and gum and works quickly upon dissolving in the mouth and being absorbed into the body.

- *Beta blockers* inhibit the effects of the hormone epinephrine (adrenaline). These medications cause the heart to beat more slowly and also lower blood pressure, thereby reducing the demand for oxygen and stress on the cardiovascular system. Beta blockers also relax blood vessels, allowing them to widen and reduce stress on the heart, and therefore the incidence of angina.

- *Calcium channel blockers* prevent calcium from entering the cells in the walls of the heart and blood vessels. They relieve angina by relaxing and widening blood vessels, lowering your blood pressure, and slowing your heart rate. These effects allow more blood to get to the heart with less work.

49. Can other conditions be mistaken for angina?

Yes, but if there is any question about the source of chest pain, seek medical attention immediately. Some of the common conditions that can be mistaken for angina include:

- Indigestion, heartburn, or acid reflux (stomach acids rising into the esophagus)

- Injury to a chest muscle, rib, or sternum
- Nerve injury in the neck or spine

Even if the source of the pain is not angina, these other causes—particularly if not previously experienced—warrant careful monitoring and medical attention if they persist or worsen.

50. How do I know if the other signs and symptoms indicate heart disease or something else?

Only a medical professional and appropriate testing can diagnose heart or cardiovascular disease. The other symptoms of heart disease—such as shortness of breath, palpitations, weakness, dizziness—can all be due to other causes. They may be relatively benign, or they may signal an important health concern. Even if not heart disease, the symptoms may indicate a different problem that requires attention. Pay attention to your body and how you feel, be aware of what is normal or expected for you, and see your doctor if you experience any of these symptoms without an apparent explanation.

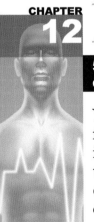

CHAPTER 12 *Diagnosis of Heart Disease*

51. How will my doctor diagnose whether I have coronary heart disease?

Your doctor will likely begin with gathering information from you about your symptoms, your risk factors (explained in detail in Part Two), and your family history. Based on this and any other information considered important, your doctor may administer any one—and frequently more than one—of the following diagnostic procedures:

- EKG (electrocardiogram)
- Cardiac stress test
- Echocardiogram

- Chest X-ray
- Coronary angiography
- Positron emission tomography (PET) scan
- Cardiac computerized tomography (CT) scan
- Electron beam computed tomography (EBCT) scan
- Cardiac magnetic resonance imaging (MRI)
- Holter monitor test
- Blood tests

52. What is an electrocardiogram (or EKG)?

An electrocardiogram (EKG) is a simple, noninvasive (outside the body) test that records the electrical impulses that pass through the chambers of the heart during their sequences of contraction and relaxation. The purpose is to detect any abnormalities in heart rhythm that suggest heart disease or other medical condition. A technician attaches electrical monitoring sensors to the skin of the chest around the heart, and the EKG apparatus detects and records the heart's electrical activity on a strip of paper. The results can help tell your doctor if:

- There is any irregularity in the strength, timing, or rhythm of your heartbeat in any area of the heart,

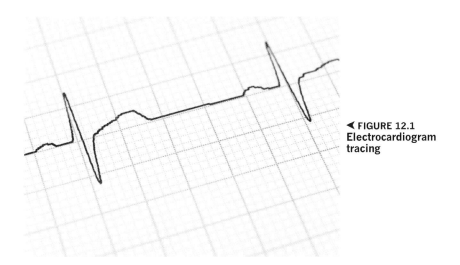

◄ FIGURE 12.1
Electrocardiogram
tracing

For a detailed animation and explanation of your heart's electrical system, go to:

ON THE WEB

http://www.nhlbi.nih.gov/health/health-topics/topics/hhw/electrical.html

- The heart has been damaged by heart disease or a heart attack, or
- There are other abnormalities of the heart.

53. What is a cardiac stress test?

In some cases, heart disease may not be immediately apparent from an EKG performed when you are at rest. In a **cardiac stress test**, you engage in controlled and increasingly vigorous exercise—typically on a treadmill or stationary bicycle—to raise your heart rate and respiration (breathing) rate. Before, during, and after the exercise, the doctor or technician will perform an EKG and monitor blood pressure, sometimes in combination with other tests. Because the heart works harder and needs more oxygen during exercise, a stress test may reveal evidence of heart disease that is not detectable at rest, including:

- Abnormalities in heart rate, rhythm, or electrical activity
- Abnormal changes in blood pressure
- Chest pain or shortness of breath

People whose physical condition prevents them from safely engaging in exercise may be given a drug that increases heart rate to simulate the effects of exercise on the heart and cardiovascular system.

54. What is an echocardiogram?

An **echocardiogram** is a noninvasive diagnostic test that uses sound waves (often called ultrasound) to produce images of the heart and its primary components—the chambers, valves, and major blood vessels that exit from the left and right ventricles. There are different types of echocardiogram technologies, such as 1-, 2-, and 3-dimensional and Doppler technology, which focuses on blood flow through the chambers and valves. Echocardiography is not typically used to detect the buildup of plaque in the coronary arteries, but rather to diagnose other types of heart problems, some of which may be evidence of coronary heart disease. An echocardiogram is used to detect:

- Congenital heart defects in the structure or function of the heart
- Disease or malfunction in the valves of the heart
- Enlargement of the heart (*cardiomyopathy*) due to thickening or weakening of the heart muscle. This condition can be evidence of cardiovascular disease
- Inflammation of the membrane around the heart (*pericarditis*)
- *Aneurysm*, or a thinning or weakening of the wall of a coronary artery or the aorta

An echocardiogram may be administered in combination with other tests, such as an EKG. There are no known health risks associated with sound wave technology, in contrast to exposure to large amounts of X-ray radiation.

55. How is a chest X-ray used to diagnose heart disease?

With the development of other more effective diagnostic tests, X-ray of the chest, heart, and lungs are no longer typically the first choice for diagnosing suspected coronary heart disease. However, an X-ray can be useful to identify abnormalities in the size or structure of the heart or the presence of fluid around the heart or in the lungs, and may be used as part of a coronary angiography test (see Question 56 below).

56. What is a coronary angiogram?

A **coronary angiogram** is a diagnostic test that is administered to detect the presence and extent of atherosclerosis (plaque buildup) in the coronary arteries. In a coronary angiogram, a special dye is injected into the coronary arteries through a procedure called cardiac catheterization.

DEFINITION

A long tube, or catheter, is inserted into a blood vessel—typically in the groin area—and gently pushed through the blood vessel until the end reaches the appropriate place in or around the heart. The special dye is released through the catheter and the dye flows through the coronary arteries. The flow of the dye can be seen on a special type of X-ray device, which is also used during the insertion of the catheter to make sure that it is in the correct location prior to releasing the dye. By following the flow of the dye through the coronary arteries, the doctor can see the presence, location, and severity of any narrowing or blockages in the arteries as well as a number of other abnormalities in the arteries.

A coronary angiogram is administered in a hospital while you are awake, often with a mild sedative to help you relax. It is a safe procedure, and most people experience little or no discomfort except some minor soreness where the catheter was inserted.

To watch an animation of a coronary angiogram procedure, visit:

ON THE WEB

http://www.youtube.com/watch?v=eTKICIpShaA

57. What is tomography, and how it is used to diagnose heart disease?

There are several different tomography technologies, but in general, **tomography** refers to the process of creating computer-generated, 3-dimensional sectional images from penetrating wave devices such as X-rays or ultrasound. When used to diagnose heart disease, the detailed images produced by tomography technology allow medical professionals to look for abnormalities and damage in the heart and coronary arteries. Tomography procedures are noninvasive but may include the intravenous administration of dye or other substances to create the images of the heart and arteries. Examples of tomography include:

- *computed (or computerized) axial tomography* (or CAT scan) is the older name for what is now most commonly called a *CT scan*. This technology uses X-rays to produce multiple images which are combined by computer to create cross-sectional views of the heart and blood vessels.

- *magnetic resonance imaging* (MRI) uses a magnetic field to position certain components of the nucleus of body cells, and radio-frequency waves and a computer to produce images. MRI technology can be combined with angiography to view the flow of blood through blood vessels.

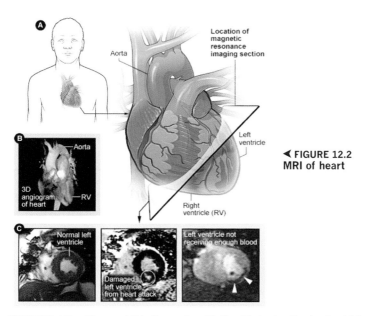

◄ FIGURE 12.2
MRI of heart

SOURCE: http://www.nhlbi.nih.gov/health/health-topics/topics/mri/show.html

• *positron emission tomography* (PET) is a nuclear imaging technique that produces 3-dimensional images of tissues—in the case of a cardiac PET, images of heart tissue. To conduct a PET, a small amount of radioactive tracer material is administered intravenously, and after allowing time for the material to reach the target area, a gamma ray camera detects the radiation and computers are used to create the images. A PET may be performed as a stress test, which, as described above, means that the heart rate is elevated through exercise or drugs to see how the heart and coronary arteries function under stress. One particular advantage of a PET scan is that it can show the degree of damage to heart tissue; for example, whether after a heart attack some heart tissue has died due to lack of oxygen from a blocked artery. Tissue that is shown to be viable may still benefit from procedures to increase blood flow to that tissue.

58. What is a Holter monitor?

A **Holter monitor** is a device that records the electrical rhythms of your heart over a period of time—typically 24 hours. Small sticky electrode patches are attached to your chest and each patch has a wire that connects to the recording device, which is carried in a pocket or a belt pouch. Essentially, a Holter monitor test is an electrocardiogram that extends over a period of time to record heart rhythm during your normal daily activities. Your doctor will ask you to carefully record all of your activities while you are wearing the monitor in order to match your activity with your heart rhythm patterns at that time. You will also be asked to note the time of any physical symptoms you experience during your activities, such as chest pain, shortness of breath, dizziness, or light-headedness. A Holter monitor test can help determine whether there are abnormal electrical rhythms or compromised blood flow to parts of the heart over a broad range of daily activities.

Yes, and they look for different clues to cardiovascular health. Here are some of the tests and what they show:

- *Homocysteine.* Homocysteine is an amino acid normally present in the body and, like other amino acids, is used by the body to make proteins. However, excessive levels of homocysteine have been linked to a higher risk of heart disease because it:

  - Can damage the lining of blood vessels and cause inflammation

  - Has been linked to atherosclerosis (plaque buildup and hardening of the arteries)

  - Has been linked to excessive clotting

A simple blood test can measure homocysteine levels. In some cases, high homocysteine levels may be caused by a dietary deficiency in folic acid (folate), vitamin B6, and vitamin B12, which help transform homocysteine into other amino acids. For people with only slightly-to-moderately elevated homocysteine levels, eating more foods rich in these vitamins or taking vitamin supplements may reduce homocysteine to more desirable levels. Following are ranges for homocysteine levels:

5–15 (micromoles/liter)	normal
15–30	moderate elevation
30–100	intermediate elevation
over 100	severely elevated

- *C-reactive protein (CRP).* C-reactive protein is a protein produced by the liver as part of a response to injury or infection, and signifies inflammation somewhere in the body. Because inflammation plays a key role in the development of atherosclerosis, a CRP analysis—done through a blood test—can be one tool in the diagnosis of heart disease. However, the presence of CRP will not tell a doctor where the

The American Heart Association does not yet recommend routine CRP screening.

inflammation is, so it cannot specifically identify coronary heart disease as the source. Because there are various reasons why someone may have noteworthy CRP levels, this test is typically only administered to people suspected of having heart disease, or who have high risk factors for heart disease. Following are heart disease risk ranges for C-reactive protein levels:

Less than 1 milligram/liter	low risk
1–3 mg/liter	average risk
Above 3mg/liter	high risk

- *Fibrinogen.* Fibrinogen is a normally occurring protein in our blood that helps blood to clot. But abnormal levels of fibrinogen may promote excessive clumping of platelets (which are largely responsible for clotting), and may exacerbate existing inflammation or injury to the walls of arteries. Many heart attacks are caused by rapidly forming clots where atherosclerosis is already present. Like C-reactive protein levels, fibrinogen levels alone cannot specifically diagnose heart or cardiovascular disease, but for people with high-risk factors for heart disease, testing fibrinogen levels can add to a medical professional's assessment of heart disease risk.

- *Lipid profile.* As we discussed in Chapter 5, a lipid profile is a blood test that will disclose total cholesterol, low-density lipoprotein (LDL, or bad) cholesterol, high-density lipoprotein (HDL, or good) cholesterol, and triglyceride levels. Unfavorable lipid profile results do not by themselves indicate heart disease, but can help your doctor assess heart disease risk when considered along with physical symptoms and other risk factors for heart disease. For lipid profile levels and correlation to heart disease risk, see Questions 11 (cholesterol) and 16 (triglycerides).

- *Apolipoprotein.* Apolipoproteins (or Apos) are specific protein molecules found in lipoproteins, including HDLs and LDLs. Apo A1 is the primary protein in HDLs (part of good cholesterol), and a low level may indicate an increased risk of heart disease. Apo B is a major protein in LDLs (part of bad cholesterol) and recent research suggests that high Apo B levels may be an even more reliable indicator of cardiovascular disease risk than high LDL cholesterol levels alone. These more advanced Apo tests are not yet generally part of a routine lipid profile, but are often performed for people with symptoms of coronary artery disease or significant risk factors for heart disease.

60. Is there a blood test that can help diagnose heart failure?

Yes. Recall that heart failure is when the heart muscle is compromised and not strong enough or not flexible enough to adequately pump blood through the body. There is now a blood test that, rather than indicate possible heart disease, has been proven to help determine whether someone has heart failure. There are two proteins (called *B-type natriuretic peptides*, or BNPs) released by damaged heart tissue to help relieve stress or overwork caused by heart failure. The levels of BNPs rise and fall as the symptoms of heart failure worsen or get better, and a doctor may take a series of BNP tests to see how heart failure is responding to drugs or other therapies.

61. Is there a test that can predict a likely heart attack?

There is a relatively new blood test that has shown a high correlation to the primary condition that precedes a heart attack, and that is therefore gaining support as a predictor of future heart attack. A heart attack is most often caused by a rupture of the plaque-covered lining of coronary arteries, which leads to the formation of a clot which in turn blocks either that artery, or another one. The cells that line coronary arteries are called endothelial cells.

Endothelial cells are believed to break off of the lining of weakening blood vessels before the lining ruptures and a clot forms that could cause a heart attack. These are called *circulating endothelial cells*, or *CECs*. The new test measures CEC levels in the blood. An abnormal level of circulating endothelial cells signals coronary artery weakness that could lead to rupture, clotting, and ultimately a heart attack. While researchers have known for years that CECs could be a predictor of heart attack, recent advances in medical technology have enabled more precise measurement of CECs, thereby enhancing the reliability of the test for future heart attack.

CASE STUDY

To see how the symptoms, diagnosis, treatment, and progression of angina and heart disease can happen in real life, consider George's experience.

Three years ago when George was in his mid-50s, he began to feel tightness in his chest and shortness of breath during his daily walk to work. It was only a mile, and he took it at a leisurely pace to enjoy the exercise and the weather, but he knew something wasn't right. Because the symptoms went away after resting at his desk when he got to work, he put it out of his mind. When it kept happening, he went to his doctor, thinking he had a chest infection.

The doctor asked about George's lifestyle, and learned that George was a pack-a-day smoker, did not pay attention to his diet, and was somewhat overweight but not obese. After listening to George's symptoms and running some tests, George's doctor ruled out a chest infection—suspecting angina instead. George was referred to a local hospital for a full cardiac examination, including an EKG, angiogram, ultrasound, cardiac enzyme assay, and lipid profile for cholesterol.

When the results came back, his doctor's preliminary diagnosis was confirmed—George had blockages in three coronary arteries ranging from 30% to 70% blocked. After discussing treatment options, George and his doctor decided to try a combination of lifestyle changes and medication to control the angina and minimize the progression of coronary heart disease, but the doctor advised George that at some point coronary bypass surgery would likely be necessary.

George was given a nitrate medication to ease the symptoms when he had an angina attack, committed to quit smoking, eat a healthier diet to lose weight, and continue with regular, moderate exercise. He did quite well not smoking, but not well at all improving his diet, which he blamed on quitting smoking and the stress of knowing he had heart disease.

A couple of months later, George had such an episode of such severe angina that he thought he had suffered a heart attack. Crushing pain in his chest radiated down his arm, and he collapsed on the sidewalk outside his office. A bystander called for an ambulance, and he was rushed to the hospital. A battery of tests disclosed that George had not suffered a heart attack, but his coronary artery disease had worsened and now all three arteries were blocked to the point that a bypass procedure was required for each of them.

George had successful surgery, and after recovering, was free of angina attacks and fully committed to lifestyle changes that would keep him healthy for a long time. He also found that with the anxiety and stress of angina attacks behind him, it was easier to make the changes necessary to stay healthy.

Adapted from CardiacMatters

Symptoms, Diagnosis, and Emergency Treatment of a Heart Attack

62. What is a heart attack?

A **heart attack**, medically known as a **myocardial infarction**, is the result of a blockage of a coronary artery that prevents oxygen-rich blood from flowing to an area of the heart.

DEFINITION

The blockage is usually caused by a clot that obstructs the flow of blood in a coronary artery that is narrowed due to the buildup of plaque—known as *atherosclerosis*, the primary type of coronary heart disease. (See Chapter 4 for a detailed discussion.) Clots can form when there is a rupture or other irregularity on the surface of layers of

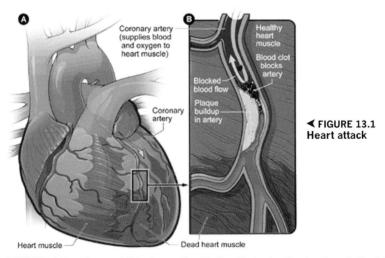

◄ FIGURE 13.1
Heart attack

SOURCE: http://www.nhlbi.nih.gov/health/health-topics/topics/heartattack/

plaque in a coronary artery, which triggers the blood's clotting response. Therefore, the buildup of plaque is the major cause of heart attack for two reasons—it narrows the coronary arteries, and it is the underlying cause of the clots that block the arteries. If the blood flow through the blocked artery is not quickly restored, the heart muscle tissue in the affected area of the heart will begin to die.

 Heart disease is the leading cause of death for both men and women in the United States. According to the CDC, every year about 785,000 Americans have a first heart attack, and another 470,000 have their second (or more) heart attack. According to the National Heart, Lung, and Blood Institute, it is estimated that there are 1.1 million heart attacks each year, and 515,000 people die from heart attacks.

63. What are the symptoms of a heart attack?

There are many different signs and symptoms of a heart attack, and not everyone feels them in the same ways. In some cases, there may be none of the common symptoms at the onset of a heart attack, or the symptoms may be very mild and not recognized as a heart attack—this is known as a "silent" heart attack. The signs and symptoms of a heart attack include:

- Pain or discomfort in the center or left side of the chest that does not go away in a few minutes. It may be sharp pain, or an uncomfortable feeling of fullness, pressure, squeezing, aching, or tightness. The pain or discomfort may come and go.
- Abnormal heart beat or heart rhythms, such as the feeling of heavy beating or palpitations.
- Shortness of breath, which may or may not be accompanied by pain or discomfort.
- Pain or discomfort in parts of the upper body, including the shoulders, arms, neck, back, jaw, teeth, or upper abdominal area.
- Dizziness, lightheadedness, or feeling faint.
- Nausea or vomiting.

- Sudden cold or clammy sweatiness.
- Lack of energy, fatigue, or sleeplessness.
- Anxiety.
- In cases of severe heart attack, some of the first symptoms may be loss of consciousness and blue discoloration of the lips, hands, or feet.
- Symptoms that resemble a stroke, such a paralysis or disorientation, more commonly seen in older people.

About 20%–30% of people suffering a heart attack do not experience chest pain. This group includes women (see Question 64 below), people older than 75, people who have heart failure or who have had a stroke, and people with a long history of insulin-dependent diabetes who may have impaired nerve sensitivity.

See the National Heart, Lung, and Blood Institute's short video on recognizing the signs of heart attack at:

ON THE WEB

http://www.nhlbi.nih.gov/health/health-topics/videos/heart-attack-warning-symptoms.html

64. Are heart attack symptoms the same for men and women?

Both men and women are susceptible to the same symptoms of a heart attack. However, studies have shown that women are more likely than men to experience symptoms other than chest pain, such as pain, aching, or discomfort in the neck, arm, or jaw, back, shoulders, or abdomen. Women are also more likely to experience dizziness, lightheadedness, sweating, nausea, vomiting, or extreme fatigue—without chest pain—than men are. Because women more often than men do not exhibit the obvious symptom of severe chest pain and the other

For a comparison of symptoms experienced by 100 men and women who had suffered heart attacks, see:

PRACTICAL TIP

http://www.webmd.com/heart-disease/news/20050218/men-vs-women-confusion-over-heart-symptoms?page=2 symptoms may be indicative of a less urgent condition, women are more likely to die of a heart attack because they may not seek immediate medical attention for the less obvious symptoms.

To watch an interview between Charlie Rose and a New York hospital cardiologist about the atypical symptoms of heart attack for women, visit:

http://www.cbsnews.com/video/watch/?id=7399673n&tag=mncol;lst;10

65. What should someone do if he or she, or another person, may be having a heart attack?

If you think you or someone else may be having a heart attack, call 911 or your local emergency number right away and request an ambulance. Response time in case of a heart attack is critical to minimizing damage to the heart—and to saving a life if the heart attack is severe. It is far better to learn after emergency treatment that the symptoms were not those of a heart attack than to delay emergency treatment for a heart attack. Emergency responders can administer time-sensitive treatment to minimize damage to the heart and alert the hospital's medical staff to what services may be required upon arrival.

While waiting for emergency help to arrive, elevate the person's feet, reassure him or her that help is on the way (this may help to reduce stress), and if possible, give them a regular aspirin dissolved in water. Aspirin is a natural blood thinner, and may help prevent further clotting.

It is critical to call for emergency medical help as soon as possible if there is a suspected heart attack. According to the National Heart, Lung, and Blood Institute, of the people who die from heart attacks, about half die within the first hour of the first symptoms, and before they reach the hospital.

66. What emergency treatment is given to someone who is believed to have had a heart attack?

Treatment begins even before a suspected heart attack patient gets to a hospital, and before the diagnosis of heart attack is confirmed. Preliminary treatment includes:

- Administration of oxygen
- Preliminary diagnostics for heart attack
- Aspirin to thin blood and reduce further clotting
- Nitroglycerin to reduce stress on the heart
- Treatment for chest pain
- Cardiopulmonary resuscitation, if required

67. How do doctors diagnose if someone has had a heart attack?

Once a patient gets to the hospital, doctors will take steps to confirm whether the person has suffered a heart attack. The diagnosis of a heart attack is made on the basis of:

1. Physical symptoms, as described in Question 63, in light of the person's health history and risk factors

2. Diagnostic procedures, typically the same ones that are used to determine the presence of coronary heart disease, including:
   - Electrocardiogram (EKG)
   - Echocardiogram
   - Coronary angiogram

3. Blood tests for substances called cardiac markers

68. What are the blood tests that can diagnose a heart attack?

When the heart muscle is damaged due to a heart attack, it releases certain substances into the blood that can be detected through a blood test. These substances are known as *serum cardiac markers* or *cardiac serum markers*. When someone is suspected to have suffered a heart attack, doctors test a blood sample for the presence of these substances, which can confirm the occurrence of a heart attack as well as its severity—how much damage the heart muscle has suffered. The primary blood tests to diagnose a heart attack are:

- *Troponin*. A troponin test is the most sensitive and specific test for myocardial (heart) damage. Up until recently, a test called the Troponin I test was considered the most reliable in diagnosing a heart attack, and it is still widely used. Now, a newer version of the troponin test—called the *highly sensitive troponin I assay*—has been developed that is believed to be even more accurate and precise in diagnosing the occurrence and severity of a heart attack. This test can be especially helpful in the case of a mild heart attack when other tests are not conclusive. Both forms of the troponin test are considered more accurate indicators of heart attack than tests for other cardiac markers and, like tests for other markers, they are generally performed multiple times following a suspected heart attack to monitor the increases and decreases in levels of marker proteins.

- *Creatine phosphokinase* (*CKP* or *CK*). Creatine phosphokinase is an enzyme contained in muscle cells that is part of a biochemical process in the production of energy. CK-MB is a particular form of CK that is found specifically in heart muscle cells. When heart muscle tissue is damaged—such as during a heart attack—CK-MB escapes from the damaged muscle cells and into the blood stream. CK and CK-MB are markers for heart attack that can be detected and measured through a blood test. The presence and level of these markers can help confirm the occurrence and severity of a heart attack. While CK tests are considered reliable, studies suggest that troponin tests are better diagnostic tools for heart attack.

- *Other tests*. There are other blood tests for possible damage to heart muscle that may be indicative of a heart attack, but they have been largely replaced by the more specific troponin and CK tests. For example, lactate dehydrogenase (LDH) is a substance released by damaged tissue and therefore may be present after a heart attack, but the cardiac form of this enzyme may not show elevated levels for a day or two after a heart attack.

69. If the diagnosis of heart attack is confirmed, what drugs will be administered?

Once medical staff have confirmed a likely heart attack, the priorities are to: (1) restore blood flow through blocked coronary arteries, (2) minimize the risk of additional blockages, and (3) reduce the strain on the heart. Initial drug treatments may include:

- "Clot busting" drugs, called *thrombolytics*, dissolve clots in the arteries to restore blood flow to affected areas of the heart. Because of the speed with which oxygen-deprived heart tissue can die, prompt administration of thrombolytics is essential to saving the patient's life in the case of a severe heart attack, and to minimizing permanent damage to the heart.

- Clot preventing drugs (sometimes called "blood thinners"), primarily *anti-platelet drugs* and *anti-coagulants*, act to inhibit the formation of new clots. Contrary to the name "blood thinner," these drugs do not actually thin the blood. Because it is platelets in the blood that clump together to form clots, these drugs work by disrupting that process. In general, anti-platelet drugs work on the clotting factor of platelets themselves, while anti-coagulants inhibit other nonplatelet chemical clotting factors that promote the clumping of platelets. Here are examples of the most commonly used clot-preventing drugs, and there are other effective drugs in both categories:

  — Anti-platelet: aspirin and clopidogrel (often sold under the name Plavix)

- Anti-coagulant: heparin and warfarin (often sold under the name Coumadin)
- Drugs to lower blood pressure and reduce strain on the heart, including *diuretics*, *beta blockers*, and *ACE inhibitors*. These are discussed in detail in Chapter 15.

70. How is coronary angioplasty used to treat a heart attack?

In addition to drug therapies, a heart attack patient may under go a procedure called **coronary angioplasty** to open or widen a blocked or narrowed coronary artery. Coronary angioplasty involves threading a thin, flexible catheter through a blood vessel to the blocked or narrowed area of a coronary artery. There is a small balloon at the tip of the catheter, which is inflated against the walls of the artery. The inflated balloon compresses the arterial plaque against the walls of the artery, widening the artery and restoring blood flow to the heart tissue.

 While some authorities estimate that up to 1 million angioplasties are performed each year, according to the Centers for Disease Control and Prevention (CDC), over 600,000 balloon coronary angioplasties were performed in the United States in 2009.

 To watch an animation of a coronary angioplasty procedure, visit:

http://www.nlm.nih.gov/medlineplus/ency/anatomyvideos/000096.htm

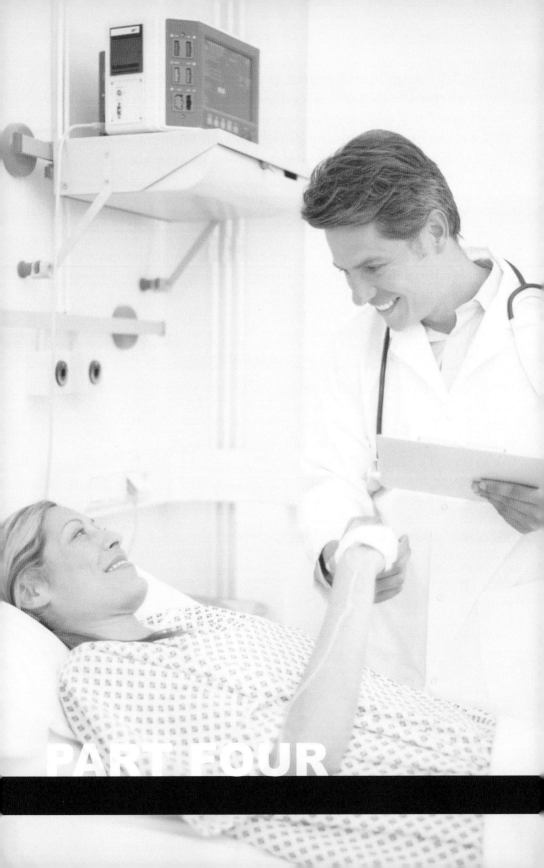

PART FOUR

Follow-Up Treatment and Recovery After a Heart Attack or Surgery

In Part Four, we will explain the implantation of heart stents to remedy blocked coronary arteries, answer questions about coronary bypass surgery, and note the use of a particular pacemaker for heart failure. Then we will progress to information about recovery from a heart attack or heart surgery, including cardiac rehabilitation and possible on-going drug therapies.

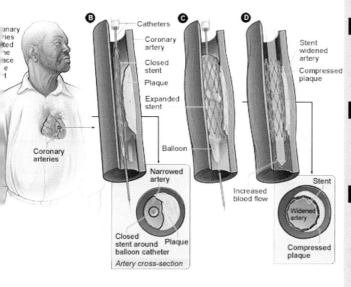

Post-Emergency Care After a Heart Attack: Stents, Bypass Surgery, and Pacemakers

CHAPTER 14

71. What medical care can someone expect after emergency treatment of a heart attack?

Following emergency treatment of a heart attack, there are a number of potential procedures and drug therapies that your doctor may recommend after a complete evaluation of your heart and coronary artery health. Medical procedures may include:

- A *heart stent*, also called a cardiac stent or coronary stent
- Other artery-clearing angioplasty procedures
- *Coronary artery bypass grafting* (CABG)
- *Biventricular pacemaker* for heart failure

Drug therapies may include the following, and they will be discussed in Chapter 15:

- Cholesterol-reducing drugs
- Blood thinners
- Blood pressure medication

Any one of these treatments, or combination of them, may also be part of the initial emergency treatment of a heart attack upon arrival at a hospital.

72. What is a heart stent?

A **heart stent** is a small expandable tube, usually made of metal mesh, that is inserted into a coronary artery to keep the artery open when it has been narrowed or blocked by plaque (atherosclerosis). The stent keeps plaque pressed against the walls of the artery, allowing blood—with its

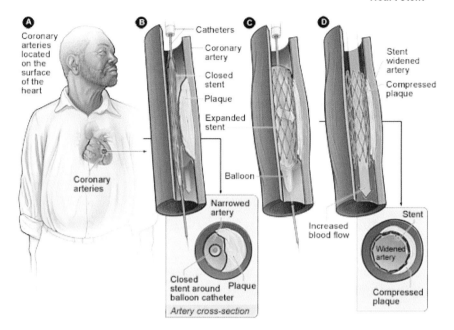

A Coronary arteries located on the surface of the heart

Coronary arteries

B Catheters

Coronary artery

Closed stent

Plaque

Expanded stent

Balloon

Narrowed artery

Closed stent around balloon catheter   Plaque

Artery cross-section

C

D Stent widened artery

Compressed plaque

Increased blood flow

Stent

Widened artery

Compressed plaque

SOURCE: http://www.nhlbi.nih.gov/health/health-topics/topics/stents/placed.html

supply of oxygen—to flow more freely to the heart tissue. A stent may also provide structural support for a weakened artery. Some stents are coated with a drug to help prevent the artery from getting blocked again—these are called *drug-eluting* stents.

73. How is a heart stent put into a coronary artery?

A heart stent is inserted into a coronary artery through a procedure called coronary angioplasty, which we discussed in Question 70. Coronary angioplasty involves the insertion of a long, flexible tube (catheter) through a blood vessel and the catheter is guided by X-ray through the blood vessels to the affected area of the heart. The stent is at the end of the catheter, and is first placed and then expanded at the location of the blockage or narrowing in the artery. Some stents are self-expanding upon placement in the artery, and others are expanded by inflating a balloon inside the stent to press it against the walls of the artery.

A heart stent procedure is considered "noninvasive" because it does not require a major incision and is performed only with local anesthesia at the site the catheter is inserted. The patient is given a mild sedative, and can generally go home shortly after the procedure or may stay in the hospital overnight for observation.

74. What are the benefits of heart stents?

Heart stents offer a number of benefits to people with coronary heart disease and who have suffered a heart attack or are at a high risk of heart attack due to blockages in coronary arteries. The benefits include:

- Immediately improved blood flow through the artery
- Relief from angina pain
- They are considered to be generally safe and effective
- Lessening of restenosis—the re-blocking of the artery over time—with drug-eluting stents coated with drugs that are intended to minimize scarring in the artery
- Less invasive procedure compared to surgical options, and does not require general anesthesia
- Lower cost compared to surgical options
- Allows resumption of normal activities soon after procedure

Some research has indicated that heart stents may not be the best treatment choice in patients with stable coronary artery disease, suggesting instead that a combination of medication and lifestyle changes are equally effective and without the risks of stents. Ask your doctor about all of the short-term and long-term benefits and risks of having a heart stent procedure.

75. Are there risks associated with heart stents?

Yes—while heart stents have helped millions of patients and are generally safe, there are some risks associated with heart stent procedures. Risks include:

- Potential injury to the artery where the catheter is inserted, or at the location where the stent is placed
- Potential formation of a blood clot at the site of the stent, leading to heart attack or stroke
- Potential formation of scar tissue at the site of the stent
- Potential adverse reaction to the contrast dye, particularly in people with pre-existing kidney disease or compromised kidney function
- Mistaken belief that a stent "cures" heart disease or eliminates the risk of future heart attack

Each of these risks is generally regarded as small, but there are occasional serious complications from cardiac catheterization and stent procedures. It is important to discuss them fully with your doctor. While your doctor may strongly recommend a stent procedure based on your medical condition, risk factors, and prognosis, ask whether a combination of medication and healthy lifestyle changes may be a viable alternative.

76. Are there other angioplasty procedures to remedy narrowed or blocked coronary arteries?

Yes. There are other types of angioplasty procedures that actually remove plaque from blocked or narrowed coronary arteries, as opposed to compressing the plaque against the artery walls with a balloon and keeping the artery open with a stent. Two primary ones are *atherectomy* and *rotational atherectomy* (or *rotoblation*). These types of procedures share the common feature of using microscopic blades, rotors, or lasers at the end of the catheter to shave off, grind off, or to vaporize the plaque from the artery walls. The plaque is either removed from the artery as part of the procedure, or the plaque is reduced to minute particles that can flow freely in the blood without posing a risk of creating further blockage until the particles are eventually eliminated by the body. These procedures are not common, and might typically be performed on someone whose plaque is very dense and hard—and therefore cannot be adequately compressed with balloon angioplasty—or who have already had angioplasty and stents and still have dangerous plaque.

77. What is bypass surgery?

Coronary bypass is the commonly used term for a medical procedure called *coronary artery bypass grafting* (CABG). In a coronary bypass procedure, a healthy blood vessel from another part of the body is attached (grafted) to the heart around the blocked artery. One end of the healthy artery is attached to the blocked coronary artery above the blockage, and the other end is attached below the blockage, allowing blood flow to "bypass" the blockage and supply blood to the affected area of the heart. It is not uncommon to have more than one bypass performed during a single surgery, which is where the terms double, triple, or quadruple bypass come from.

According to a study published in the May 4, 2011 issue of the *JAMA*, the number of coronary bypass surgeries dropped substantially between 2001 and 2008, reflecting our healthier lifestyles, improved management of heart disease risk factors, and advances in less invasive angioplasty and stent procedures.

78. How is a coronary bypass procedure performed?

Traditional coronary bypass surgery—while common, considered safe, and offering proven beneficial results—is major open-heart surgery. Emergency bypass surgery is sometimes performed following a heart attack, but most often it is scheduled in advance after other options, such as lifestyle changes, medication, and angioplasty have not adequately remedied severe cardiovascular disease and the risk of heart attack is high. If you and your doctor determine that you will have coronary bypass surgery, well prior to the surgery, you would:

- Have a series of diagnostic tests to confirm that the surgery is necessary and offers a favorable outcome,

- Be given instructions on diet and physical activities, and

- Be given instructions on the use of any existing medications you're taking, or new ones that may be prescribed in advance of the surgery.

Coronary bypass is performed under general anesthesia. During the surgery, the chest is opened through the *sternum* (breastbone) to expose the heart and the surgeon confirms the location of one or more blocked arteries that will be the subject of the bypass. A healthy blood vessel may either be removed from another part of the body— often the leg—or frequently the surgeon will use a blood vessel in the chest called the *internal mammary artery* as the source of the new blood flow because it is already connected to an oxygen-rich supply of blood. The source of the blood vessels to be used for the bypass depends on the number and location of blocked arteries. During traditional coronary bypass surgery, a drug is given to stop the heart, and a heart-lung bypass machine is used to keep oxygenated blood circulating through the body during surgery. This type of bypass surgery is called *on-pump* surgery and allows the surgeon to perform the grafting procedures on a heart that is not moving. After the surgeon attaches the healthy blood vessel above and below the blockage in the diseased artery, blood will start flowing through the new blood vessel, supplying oxygen and nutrients to the affected area of the heart. The heart-lung machine will be turned off, and the heart may start beating on its own. If it doesn't (and this is common), the surgeon will re-start the heart with a mild electric shock. The surgeon will use surgical wire to close the sternum, and the entrance wound on the chest will be sutured closed.

ON THE WEB

To watch a short video about heart disease and treatment, including excerpts of an actual heart bypass performed by Dr. Mehmet Oz, visit:

http://www.thevisualmd.com/health_centers/cardiovascular_health/coronary_bypass_surgery/what_is_coronary_bypass_surgery_video

79. Are there other types of coronary bypass surgery?

Yes. Sometimes the heart is kept beating during an open-heart bypass operation and the heart-lung machine is not used—this is called *off-pump* surgery. In this procedure, the surgeon will use special equipment to keep the parts of the heart still while the grafted blood vessels are being attached. There is also a newer advancement in bypass surgery called *minimally invasive direct coronary bypass surgery* (MIDCAB or MIDCABG). In this type of bypass surgery, rather than opening the chest cavity, small incisions are made in the chest, the chest muscles are separated, and a small section of rib cartilage is removed to allow access to the affected area of the heart. The bypass graft is performed through these incisions, often with the aid of robotics and imaging technology. The heart-lung machine is not used in this operation. MIDCABG is usually used only when the artery to which the grafted blood vessel will be attached is located on the front of the heart where it can be reached through the smaller, localized incisions. The benefits of this procedure are reduced risk of infection, less bleeding, and decreased hospital stay and recovery time.

80. What are the risks of coronary bypass surgery?

While coronary bypass surgery has improved—and saved—many lives, there are risks involved. Some of the risks are common to any major surgery, including:

- Adverse reactions to anesthesia
- Infection and bleeding at the site of the incision
- Fever and pain
- Blood clots leading to heart attack or stroke
- Thick scarring
- Rarely, death

Additionally, there are risks specific to cardiac bypass surgery, including:

- Temporary neurocognitive impairment and mood disorders which may include depression, memory loss, loss of mental clarity or confusion, and lack of concentration. These issues are more frequently seen in women and in older patients, and often improve after several months.

- Heart arrhythmias or heart attack.
- Impaired healing of the sternum.
- Persistent minor fever and chest pain (post pericardiotomy syndrome, which can occur after surgical incision of the pericardium—the membrane that surrounds the heart).
- Kidney failure.

Complications from bypass surgery are more likely in people with other medical conditions, such as diabetes, kidney disease, circulatory problems, or obesity, or who have had open-heart surgery in the past. As you should with any important medical decision, discuss with your doctor the benefits and risks of coronary bypass surgery. For people with life-threatening coronary heart disease, bypass surgery is often the best—and perhaps the only—choice.

81. What is the recovery process from coronary bypass?

Coronary bypass provides immediate relief from the dangers of blocked arteries by restoring blood flow to the heart. But the operation is major surgery and full recovery is a gradual process. After the surgery, you will likely remain in the hospital's Intensive Care Unit (ICU) for a few days during which time doctors and staff will:

- Attach you to equipment that will monitor your heart and lung function, oxygen levels, blood pressure, and other vital signs
- Monitor the surgical sites for infection and healing, and may place a tube in your chest to drain the surgical wound
- Insert an intravenous line to administer fluids and medication to ease the strain on the heart
- Insert a urinary catheter so you can rest in bed

When you are ready to go home, your medical team will provide you with instructions on how to continue your recovery and optimize the results of your bypass, including:

- Visiting nurse or other home health care assistance
- Caring for your surgical wounds, and how to identify possible infection
- Any medication that may be required, for example to control blood pressure, reduce the heart's workload, or to lower cholesterol levels
- Physical activities such as returning to work, driving, sexual activity, exercise, and cardiac rehabilitation
- Managing any post-operative side-effects you may experience such as pain, swelling, or other discomfort; psychological or cognitive issues; fatigue, problems sleeping, or constipation
- Diet and nutrition

Bypass surgery does not cure coronary artery disease or eliminate the risk of future heart attack. In order to maintain the full benefits of your bypass procedure, you must continue to manage the risk factors that caused coronary artery disease in the first place.

NOTE

It may take several weeks to start feeling better after bypass surgery, and complete recovery may take 3–6 months depending on your overall health and the extensiveness of the surgery.

82. When might a pacemaker be used in someone with coronary heart disease?

We discussed in Chapters 1 and 2 the flow of blood through the chambers of the heart, to and from the lungs, and through the body. The ability of the heart to effectively pump blood depends on the proper sequence and rhythm of the contractions of the chambers of the heart. The sequence and rhythm are controlled by the heart's electrical system, and if the system isn't working as it should, doctors may insert a pacemaker—a small device that sends out electrical impulses to regulate the rhythm of the heart's contractions. A pacemaker is usually placed under the skin of the chest or abdomen.

Pacemakers are typically used to regulate irregular heart rhythms (called *arrhythmias*) such as beating too fast (*tachycardia*), too slow (*bradycardia*), quivering weakly rather than beating (*fibrillation*), and other rhythm problems. However, there is a particular pacemaker that may be used in people with heart failure, where the heart is not strong enough or flexible enough to adequately pump blood. In a healthy heart, the left and right ventricles contract at the same time. In someone with heart failure, the ventricles may not contract at the same time, preventing the heart from pumping strongly enough to push blood through the body. A *biventricular pacemaker* ensures that the ventricles contract at the same time— called *biventricular pacing*, or *cardiac resynchronization therapy*. A biventricular pacemaker may be recommended for people who continue to have severe symptoms of heart failure even with medication and other therapies.

Recovery from Heart Attack or Heart Surgery; Cardiac Rehabilitation

83. What is the recovery process and timetable after a heart attack or heart surgery?

Full recovery after a heart attack or heart surgery can be a lengthy and gradual process. Your body has been through a traumatic event. For the first couple of weeks, you would be mostly resting, healing from any surgical procedures, and getting your strength back. If you don't encounter any complications, typically you would start feeling better in 4 to 6 weeks, during which time you can start resuming some of your normal low-exertion activities, such as:

- Walking
- Climbing stairs in your home
- Food shopping
- Cooking
- Riding in a car
- Attending religious services or entertainment events
- Light therapeutic exercises if recommended by your doctor

If you are recovering from a mild heart attack and did not have any surgical procedures, your doctor will likely permit you to get back to most nonstrenuous activities sooner—sometimes within a couple of weeks. During this time, you will likely be engaged in a cardiac rehabilitation program, which we discuss in Questions 89 and 90.

Full recovery can take anywhere between 3 and 6 months. During that time, you will increase the duration and intensity of your exercises for cardiac rehabilitation, and be able to progressively engage in your usual activities.

84. When can I go back to work?

Of course, that depends on the severity of your heart attack or extensiveness of your surgery, and what type of work you do. But in general, if your work does not involve lifting objects or other physical activity, experts range from 4–12 weeks to return to work, and perhaps sooner if you are able to work part-time. You could do work-related things at home—such as phone calls, email, or computer work—as soon as you feel up to it.

85. When can I start driving?

If you are recovering from a heart attack or minimally invasive surgery, your doctor can tell you when it is safe for you to drive depending on the extent of the heart attack or procedure, the absence of any complications, and the risk of fatigue, impaired reflexes, and reaction time due to the effects of medications you may be taking. A common range would be 2–6 weeks. In addition to these considerations, if you have had open-heart surgery, you need additional time to permit your chest incision and sternum to heal. For your safety and that of others, you should wait until your condition has been stable for a week or so before you drive.

86. What about air travel?

Ask your doctor when it is OK to travel by air. When it is, here are some things to remember:

- Tell your doctor if you will be travelling to high altitudes (the air is thinner and puts more stress on your heart and cardiovascular system) or to places that may be very hot or cold
- Make sure you have all of your medications in a carry-on bag
- Give yourself extra time to avoid rushing—and stress
- Avoid carrying heavy luggage
- If you are on a long flight, get up to stretch and move around periodically
- Consider travel insurance in case you cannot make the trip

87. When can I start having sex?

Assuming you have not been experiencing chest pain or other complications, most people can resume sexual activity within a few weeks. The level of exertion is similar to walking up two flights of stairs. Here are some things to remember:

- There are both physical and emotional aspects to sexual activity. Talk with your doctor about whether you're physically healthy enough to have sex, and if you have any questions or concerns. Be open with your partner about how you're feeling physically and emotionally.

- Apprehension about whether your heart is healthy enough, and whether you are capable of your usual experience, are completely normal. These feelings may temporarily interfere with your getting back to "your old self," so be patient.

- Your body is still recovering, and you may fatigue more quickly.

- Recovery from heart attack or surgery, as well as several types of medications prescribed for heart patients, can diminish your interest in sex, arousal, and performance. This is also normal. Talk with your doctor about possible causes and remedies.

- Certain drugs that are prescribed for men to enable sexual intercourse can affect blood pressure and cause heart arrhythmias, especially when combined with medication often prescribed for heart patients. Do not take any medication without first consulting your doctor.

- If you experience pain or other abnormal symptoms, contact your doctor.

To read *What to Expect after Heart Surgery* from the Society of Thoracic Surgeons, visit:

PRACTICAL TIP

http://www.sts.org/sites/default/files/documents/pdf/whattoexpect.pdf

Most people who have had a heart attack or heart surgery can return to their usual intimacy. Your doctor can help with any medical issues.

88. Are there psychological aspects to recovering from a major heart event?

Absolutely, and recognizing and dealing with the psychological aspects is very important to both your recovery and your long-term health and quality of life. Research has shown that a significant percentage of people who have had heart surgery experience short-term—and sometimes long-term—anxiety, sadness, and depression, and the numbers are even greater for people who have suffered a heart attack. Some of the reasons for these feelings or mood issues include:

- Fear of another heart attack
- Fear of dying
- Adjusting to lifestyle changes
- Grief over the loss of health
- Feelings that you have become a burden to others

In fact, recent research indicates that some heart attack survivors experience symptoms of post-traumatic stress disorder (PTSD), which we often hear of in connection with combat veterans, rape or assault victims, and emergency responders, such as the first responders to the Sept 11th terrorist attacks. In heart attack patients, PTSD symptoms can include flashbacks to their heart attack, nightmares, and severe anxiety.

Almost everyone who has gone through a major heart event like heart attack or surgery has temporary feelings of sadness. This is normal, and should resolve relatively soon as you improve in recovery, start feeling better and experiencing the benefits of your rehabilitation, and get back to your normal activities. But if untreated, debilitating anxiety, depression, and symptoms of PTSD can:

- Interfere with your motivation and dedication to your cardiac rehabilitation efforts
- Diminish your quality of life and well being
- Raise your blood pressure
- Compromise your immune system
- Cause cardiac arrhythmias

 Studies have shown that heart attack survivors who suffer from severe depression, anxiety, or symptoms of PTSD are substantially more likely to suffer another heart attack or to die from heart disease related causes than those who do not.

To read more about the symptoms, effects, and treatment of anxiety, depression, and PTSD after a major heart event, visit:

http://www.hearthealthywomen.org/treatment-and-recovery/mental-recovery-after-a-heart-attack-or-procedure/mental-recovery.html

and

http://my.clevelandclinic.org/heart/prevention/stress/depressionandheart.aspx

PRACTICAL TIP

If you have any questions about whether what you're feeling as you recover from heart attack or heart surgery is normal, talk to your doctor. This is as important as physical rehabilitation.

89. What is cardiac rehabilitation?

Cardiac rehabilitation (rehab) is a multi-faceted recovery program for people who:

- Have recently had a heart attack,
- Have recently had heart surgery or a procedure such as coronary angioplasty or stent placement, or
- Suffer from heart failure.

Cardiac rehab programs are structured and supervised by your medical team of doctors and nurses, and may also include physical or exercise therapists, nutrition specialists or dieticians, and counselors to support the emotional and psychological aspects of recovery. Depending on your particular circumstances, needs, and limitations, a rehab program might consist of all or some combination of the following:

- A physical exam and medical tests, such as electrocardiogram, blood pressure, blood sugar, and lipid profile (for cholesterol and triglycerides), and an assessment of any medications you're taking, both for heart disease and for any other reason
- Exercise therapy to strengthen your heart and cardiovascular system

- Weight management to reduce the physical stress on your heart
- If you smoke, smoking cessation assistance
- Heart-healthy dietary education
- Helping you manage other medical conditions related to your heart health, such as diabetes
- Counseling support to help you stay on track to meet your goals

Your doctor should strongly encourage you to continue any cardiac rehab that you may have started in the hospital after a heart attack or surgery. Cardiac rehab may also be appropriate if you have symptoms of heart failure that are not responding to drug or other therapies.

90. Why is cardiac rehabilitation important?

Studies have shown that people who have had a heart attack and do not go through cardiac rehab are more likely to have another one within a shorter period of time than people who do. After a heart attack or heart surgery, you need to re-strengthen and re-condition your heart and cardiovascular system. And for long-term health, a cardiac rehab program can help you understand the risk factors that caused coronary heart disease in the first place, and teach you how to change any lifestyle habits or routines that contributed to your risk factors.

CHAPTER

On-Going Drug Therapies 16

91. What kind of drugs might be prescribed to manage the causes or consequences of coronary heart disease?

As we have briefly mentioned, there are different types of medications that are used to manage certain risk factors for, and adverse effects of, coronary heart disease. In this chapter we will take a closer look at drugs that are used to manage medical conditions that contribute to or result from heart disease, and which are often prescribed following a heart attack. The primary ones include:

- Cholesterol reducing medicines
- Blood pressure medicines
- Blood thinners (anti-clotting drugs)
- Antiarrhythmic medicines

92. I've heard of statins. What are they? Are other drugs prescribed to reduce high cholesterol?

Statins are one type of drug that is used to lower high cholesterol.

DEFINITION

Recall from Chapter 5 that there are two main types of cholesterol. High-density lipoprotein (HDL) cholesterol is good cholesterol, and protects the coronary arteries from the buildup of dangerous plaque. Low-density lipoprotein (LDL) cholesterol is bad cholesterol, and contributes to the buildup of artery-clogging plaque. Therefore, high levels of LDL cholesterol can be a significant risk factor for heart disease. There are 5 main drug therapies to control cholesterol, including:

1. *Statins.* Statins work by inhibiting the action of a liver enzyme that is required for the liver's production of cholesterol. Statins can lower LDL cholesterol and triglyceride levels, preventing or slowing the accumulation of plaque in the coronary arteries. Statins may also help to reduce the amount of plaque that has already developed in the arteries. Finally, statins may slightly raise HDL levels, which helps to fight the accumulation of arterial plaque. There are several types of statins, including a few of the well-known ones such as Lipitor (atorvastatin), Crestor (rosuvastatin), Zocor (simvastatin), Pravachol (pravastatin), Altocor and Mevacor (lovastatin), and Lescol (fluvastatin).

Statins have been proven to be very effective in reducing cholesterol in millions of people with coronary artery disease and people who have already suffered a heart attack, and most people tolerate statins without problems. But a small percentage of patients experience side effects from taking statins, some of which are potentially serious. Side effects that have been observed include:

— Liver problems, and the United States Food and Drug Administration (FDA) recommends that your doctor perform liver enzyme tests before you start on statins as a benchmark for comparison in case you experience symptoms of liver dysfunction. Your doctor will explain the symptoms that you should report to him or her, and may repeat the liver enzyme tests as appropriate.

— Serious muscle problems of different types that can cause pain, tenderness, weakness, or inflammation. In severe cases, statins can cause muscle tissue to break down, releasing a protein into the body that can cause kidney damage by making the kidneys work too hard to metabolize the protein. In extremely rare cases, this condition can ultimately lead to kidney failure and death.

— The FDA recently issued a release requiring statin labels to warn of possible, but rare, memory and cognitive problems associated with statin use, as well as a small risk of increased blood sugar levels and developing Type 2 diabetes.

— More common and less serious side effects can include headache, nausea and intestinal upset (cramping, bloating, gas, constipation, or diarrhea), muscle or joint aches, and difficulty sleeping.

To read the full (one-page) FDA Release of February 28, 2012 that explains the changes to statin labeling, and which includes helpful links to other FDA information about statins, see:

http://www.fda.gov/NewsEvents/Newsroom/PressAnnouncements/ucm293623.htm

Most of the symptoms eventually go away if you stop taking the medication, although the rare and most severe side effects can present lasting problems. You should not stop taking a medication without first consulting the doctor that prescribed it for you.

2. *Niacin (nicotinic acid).* Niacin is one of the B-complex vitamins and it serves a number of important functions in the body, such as turning carbohydrates into energy and supporting the health of digestion, nervous system, eyes, and skin. Niacin is often part of a daily vitamin supplement, though it is readily available through a balanced diet. In high doses—much higher than you could get from diet alone—niacin has been shown to boost HDL (good) cholesterol, which promotes cardiovascular health by taking away excess LDL (bad) cholesterol. Niacin may also reduce LDL cholesterol and triglycerides, both of which contribute to cardiovascular disease.

   Niacin in high doses is often prescribed along with statins, under names such as Niaspan, Niacor, and Slo-Niacin. However, while the effectiveness of niacin in improving cholesterol levels is widely accepted, there is some research that suggests that the combination of niacin and statins is no more effective than either drug alone. And high doses of niacin may increase blood sugar in some people, and is not recommended for people with high blood sugar or diabetes. There can be other side effects that may make high doses of niacin inappropriate for some people.

3. *Bile acid sequestrants.* Bile acid sequestrants work by binding bile acids (used in the digestion process) in the intestine, resulting in the bile acids being excreted by the body. The liver uses cholesterol to make and replenish the supply of bile acids, thereby reducing cholesterol levels—specifically LDL cholesterol—in the blood and preventing it from building up as plaque in the coronary arteries. Bile

acid sequestrants may be prescribed in conjunction with statins. The most common side effect of taking bile acid sequestrants is intestinal upset, primarily constipation.

4. *Fibrates.* Fibrates work primarily to reduce triglyceride levels, total cholesterol, and raise HDL (good) cholesterol, but there is no strong evidence that fibrates effectively reduce LDL (bad) cholesterol. Fibrates may be indicated for people with high triglyceride levels, or for the small percentage of people for whom statins do not work, or who experience dangerous side effects.

5. *Cholesterol absorption inhibitors.* Cholesterol absorption inhibitors (CAIs) are the most recent development in cholesterol-lowering drugs. As the name suggests, they work by inhibiting the absorption of cholesterol in the small intestine, which reduces the body's total cholesterol. While CAIs may be prescribed alone, they are more often used in combination with statins. The only CAI currently on the market is ezetimibe, sold under the brand name Zetia in the United States. The combination of ezetimibe and the simvastatin form of statin (sold as Zocor) is sold under the trade name Vytorin.

 PRACTICAL TIP To read the National Institutes of Health publication *High Blood Cholesterol: What You Need to Know*, visit:

http://www.nhlbi.nih.gov/health/public/heart/chol/wyntk.pdf

93. What kind of blood pressure medications might be prescribed for me?

We discussed in Chapter 6 what it means to have high blood pressure and why it is a risk factor for heart disease. For the same reasons, it is important for anyone with heart disease or who has had a heart attack to maintain their blood pressure at healthy levels. There are several types of blood pressure lowering drugs that are prescribed for people living with heart disease to reduce stress on the coronary arteries and ease the workload of the heart. Here is an explanation of the main categories of blood pressure drugs and what they do or how they work.

1. *Alpha blockers (alpha-adrenergic antagonists).* Alpha blockers work by interfering with the process by which certain muscles and blood vessels tighten, allowing them to relax, and in the case of blood vessels, remain open and permit greater blood flow. Alpha blockers are used to treat a number of medical conditions, and are not typically used alone to control blood pressure.

2. *Angiotensin converting enzyme (ACE) inhibitors.* ACE inhibitors work by inhibiting the production of a hormone called angiotensin that constricts the blood vessels (a condition called vasoconstriction). Inhibiting angiotensin production allows the blood vessels to widen, or dilate, which in turn allows blood to flow more easily, lowering blood pressure.

3. *Angiotensin II receptor blockers (ARBs).* Similar to ACE inhibitors, ARBs inhibit the vasoconstriction effect of angiotensin, but ARBs work by blocking the effect of angiotensin rather than inhibiting its actual production.

4. *Beta blockers.* Beta blockers inhibit the effect of the hormone adrenaline on the heart, slowing the heart rate, reducing its demand for oxygen, and causing the heart to beat with less force. These effects lower blood pressure and lower the stress on the heart and coronary arteries.

5. *Calcium channel blockers.* Calcium channel blockers work by disrupting the supply of calcium to the cells of the heart muscle and blood vessels that facilitate contraction. The result is less forceful contractions of the heart, relaxation of the arteries, and lower blood pressure. In addition to lowering blood pressure, some calcium channel blockers can also slow the

heart rate, further reducing stress on the heart and coronary arteries.

6. *Diuretics.* Sometimes known as "water pills," diuretics increase the kidneys' production of urine to eliminate excess water and sodium from the body. Lowering the volume of fluid in the blood vessels lowers the blood pressure and reduces the heart's workload. There are several types of diuretics, and some are used primarily to lower blood pressure, while others are more often prescribed for other purposes, such as to relieve the effects of heart failure.

7. *Renin inhibitors.* Renin is an enzyme that acts as the initial catalyst in the process by which angiotensins cause vasoconstriction—the constriction of blood vessels. While the role of renin in this process has been known for many years, only recently have researchers been able to develop an effective class of drugs known as *direct renin inhibitors* for use in lowering blood pressure by blocking renin's role in vasoconstriction.

8. *Vasodilators.* Vasodilators work by relaxing the muscle cells of the walls of blood vessels, allowing the blood vessels to open—dilate—and blood to flow through them more easily, thus lowering blood pressure.

The most commonly prescribed blood pressure medicines are ACE inhibitors, beta blockers, calcium channel blockers, and diuretics. Different classes of blood pressure medications are sometimes used in combination, either in one pill or by taking more than one. Blood pressure drugs all have side effects—some potentially more serious than others—and you should discuss them with your doctor. But because high blood pressure is such a significant contributor to heart and coronary artery disease, medication is necessary if diet, exercise, and other lifestyle measures are not able to control it. Your doctor's recommendation of which medication you should take will depend on a variety of factors, such as how high your blood pressure is, your specific health issues and other conditions you may have, other medications you are taking, and the potential side effects.

94. Might I have to take blood thinners?

As we've discussed, most heart attacks from coronary heart disease are caused by clots that originate in the plaque in the lining of coronary arteries. The clots break off from the plaque, and block either that coronary artery or another one. Even if you have not had a heart attack, if your doctor believes that you are at risk of clots and heart attack, he or she may prescribe a blood thinner—an anti-clotting drug—to reduce the risk of clots. And if you have had a heart attack, it is very likely that you will be given a blood thinner. We explained in Question 69 the two main types of anti-clotting drugs: anti-platelet drugs (such as aspirin and clopidogrel), and anti-coagulants (most commonly warfarin). Aspirin is an effective, readily available anti-clotting agent, and it is very common for health professionals to recommend taking a low-dose aspirin every day for anyone at risk of heart disease, and for almost everyone who has already had a heart attack. But always talk with your doctor before you take any medication. There may be reasons why this common therapy would not be appropriate for you, such as adverse interaction with other medications you're taking, or other medical conditions you have.

95. What are antiarrhythmia drugs?

Sometimes as a result of heart disease, heart attack, or after heart surgery, the heart is susceptible to abnormalities in heart rhythm—known as arrhythmias. This can mean that the heart beats too fast, or too slowly, or that there are abnormalities in the timing, strength, or sequence of the contractions of the chambers of the heart—the atria and the ventricles. These contractions are all controlled by the impulses produced by the heart's electrical system. The electrical system depends, in part, on the action of specific elements that carry or transfer the heart's electrical charges—these elements are called *electrolytes*. Heart arrhythmias due to heart disease are generally treated with antiarrhythmia drugs. There are 5 main types of antiarrhythmia drugs, including:

1. Drugs that act on sodium, an electrolyte

2. Drugs that act on potassium, an electrolyte

3. Drugs that act on calcium, an electrolyte

4. Drugs that suppress the heart's reaction to adrenaline (these are the beta blockers we discussed in connection with blood pressure)

5. Drugs that act in other ways

There are several different and specific types of heart arrhythmias—some affect the atria, some the ventricles, and others the nodes that control the electrical impulses— and the choice of antiarrhythmia drug will depend on the precise nature and severity of a person's heart arrhythmia.

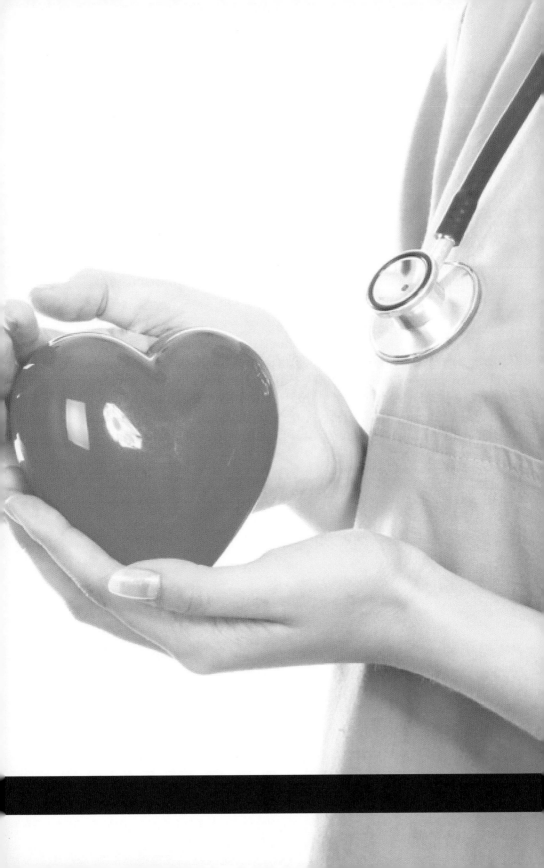

Three Keys to Heart-Healthy Living

In Part Five, we will take a detailed look at three keys to heart-healthy living. We'll start with why it is so important not to smoke, strategies for quitting, and what you can expect during the process. We will then move on to the effect of stress on cardiovascular health, types of stress, and strategies to manage it and reduce its adverse consequences. Finally, we will take an in-depth look at diet and nutrition, including weight management and two of the key dietary factors in heart health—fats and carbohydrates.

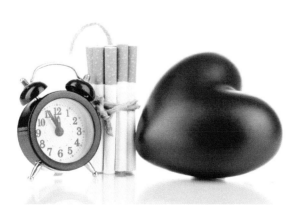

CHAPTER 17
Quitting Smoking

CHAPTER 18
Managing Stress

CHAPTER 19
Diet and Nutrition

17 *Quitting Smoking*

96. If I've had a heart attack, heart surgery, or been diagnosed with coronary heart disease, how can I work toward being the healthiest I can be?

In Part Two, we discussed the most prevalent factors that cause or contribute to heart disease, including:

- High cholesterol and triglycerides
- High blood pressure (hypertension)
- Diabetes or pre-diabetes
- Obesity
- Smoking/use of oral tobacco products
- Lack of physical activity and exercise
- Excessive alcohol consumption
- Unhealthy diet
- Family history of heart disease
- Stress

Whether you are recovering from a heart attack or heart surgery, or have been diagnosed with heart disease, it is critical that you incorporate into your lifestyle heart-healthy habits that eliminate—or reduce as much as possible—the effects of the risk factors that caused your heart disease. Neither recovery from heart attack, nor undergoing a noninvasive procedure such as angioplasty,

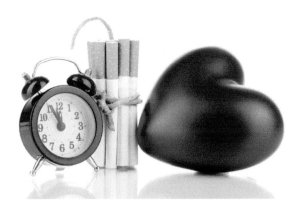

nor coronary bypass surgery will have cured your heart disease. In order to maximize the benefits of whatever therapies or procedures you've had so far, you need to be vigilant in eliminating or controlling the things that put you at risk of heart disease. In this chapter, we are going to focus more closely on quitting smoking.

97. Why should I quit smoking?

We noted in Chapter 9 many reasons why smoking is one of the highest risk factors for heart disease, including:

- Smoking increases LDL (bad) cholesterol
- Smoking increases the build up of plaque in the arteries
- Smoking increases clotting
- Smoking lowers HDL (good) cholesterol
- Smoking damages the lining of blood vessels (endothelium)
- Smoking temporarily increases blood pressure and heart rate
- Smoking can cause spasms in the coronary arteries

Smoking also reduces the amount of oxygen in the blood, which diminishes the supply to the heart tissue and reduces your tolerance for exercise. Although we are focusing in this book on heart and cardiovascular health, it is equally important to remember that smoking:

- Is the leading cause of lung cancer
- Increases the risk of cancer of the mouth, throat, esophagus, kidneys, and pancreas
- Is the leading cause of chronic obstructive pulmonary disease (COPD), primarily emphysema and chronic bronchitis

According to the American Heart Association, smoking is the most important preventable cause of premature death in the United States. The Centers for Disease Control estimates that smoking contributes to over 440,000 deaths per year.

- Increases the risk of stroke
- Is associated with lower bone density in post-menopausal women, increasing the potential for hip and other bone fracture

98. Why is it so hard to quit?

Quitting smoking can be difficult, primarily because of the multiple addictive properties of nicotine. Nicotine itself is an addictive stimulant. But research also suggests that nicotine causes increased levels of dopamine, a powerful neurotransmitter that plays a large part in the reward and pleasure responses in the brain. The addictive properties of nicotine have been likened to those of heroin and cocaine. But with dedication and perseverance—and the promise of good heart health—people *do* quit.

99. What are some strategies that give me the best chance of quitting?

First, you have to decide if you are going to quit by gradually reducing your smoking until you no longer smoke at all, or by simply quitting all smoking "cold turkey" starting on some day that you designate as your quitting day. Studies seem mixed on whether one strategy is clearly more effective than the other. However, if you have heart disease, or have had a heart attack or heart surgery, quitting all at once as soon as possible is the better choice. The effects of any amount of smoking are detrimental to heart health, and your doctor will likely tell you to quit smoking—if not yesterday, then today! So assuming you want to quit smoking all at once, here are some strategies and tips on how to succeed.

1. Be committed. Remind yourself of all of the reasons you want to quit—for your health, your enjoyment of life, your loved ones. . . anything that will help you sustain your motivation.

2. Remove all smoking materials from your home, car, or anywhere you typically smoke. This includes cigarettes, matches and lighters, and ashtrays. If

smoking materials are not at hand when you have the urge to smoke, you have a much better chance of overcoming the craving, which is strongest at the times you would normally smoke. And by removing the materials, you are reminding yourself of your commitment.

3. Be cognizant of your smoking "triggers." This means recognizing the times or circumstances that you are typically most likely to smoke; for example, with your morning coffee, when you feel stress, when you're bored, after a meal, when you're with friends who smoke, with an alcoholic beverage after work, or before going to bed. Addiction to smoking is both physical and psychological, and by being mindful of your triggers you can anticipate when your desire to smoke is likely to be the strongest, and you can be prepared.

4. Make a plan to deal with your triggers. The strongest initial craving passes quickly—often within a few minutes. Have a glass of water, chew a piece of gum, eat a piece of fruit, take a walk, call a friend, read the newspaper, a magazine, or a book, tackle a project around the house, engage in any hobbies or activities you enjoy—anything to interrupt the immediate craving when you would typically smoke.

5. Tell your family and friends that you are quitting and enlist their support. If they are smokers, ask them not to smoke around you.

6. Hopefully you will have started on a program of exercise or other physical activity to improve your heart health. When you get the urge to smoke, do your exercises, or head out to the gym or health club. Remind yourself that smoking interferes with your cardiovascular conditioning.

7. Talk with your doctor about smoking cessation aids. Products currently on the market include:

   — Nicotine patches, gum, lozenges, inhalers, and nasal sprays. While they still contain nicotine, they eliminate the intake of the other harmful chemicals of tobacco products, and won't interfere with the oxygen levels in your blood like smoking does. They also allow you to taper off of nicotine in controlled doses. Do not replace smoking with smokeless tobacco such as chewing tobacco.

— The United States Food and Drug Administration (FDA) has approved two prescription smoking cessation drugs. One is sold under the name Chantix, and the other under the name Zyban. They work by acting on how the brain reacts to nicotine. While these drugs may be effective for some people to help them quit smoking, the FDA requires both drugs to carry strong warnings of possible side severe effects.

— A new device is currently being tested that is shaped like a cigarette, delivers a nicotine vapor when inhaled, and most closely replicates the sensation of cigarette smoking compared to products currently on the market. As of this writing, this device has not yet received FDA approval.

8. Explore whether there are support groups in your area where you can meet and talk with other people who are quitting smoking. Some people benefit from sharing their experience with others who are also going through the same thing and understand the challenges. You may also learn techniques to help you more effectively deal with your triggers.

9. Some health-related organizations offer educational materials to help people who are quitting smoking, and many of them are free. For example, you can request an educational brochure from the American Heart Association at: http://www.heart.org/HEARTORG/General/Quit-Smoking-for-Good_UCM_310564_Article.jsp

10. Finally, envision yourself as a nonsmoker rather than a smoker who is trying to quit.

100. I've heard about "withdrawal." What should I expect?

Quitting smoking involves breaking your body's addiction to nicotine, and most people do experience physiological effects to some degree. The severity of the withdrawal effects depends mostly on how long you smoked and how much you smoked. Symptoms of nicotine withdrawal can include:

- Irritability or impatience
- Difficulty concentrating
- Anxiety
- Restlessness
- Difficulty sleeping
- Constipation

These symptoms typically subside in 10–14 days, perhaps longer if you were a long-term heavy smoker. However the urge to smoke can continue to last for an indefinite time— the brain has become acclimated to the physiological effects of nicotine. When you feel the urge to smoke, focus on all of the progress you've made, the health benefits you've already rewarded yourself with for however long you have not smoked, and give yourself credit for your dedication to your goals. They're worth the effort.

101. What if I slip and smoke again?

Most people trying to quit smoking relapse before they successfully quit for good—some estimates range up to 75%. In fact, many people relapse more than once, and it is not uncommon to try two or three, or even more times. If you are truly committed to quitting, don't be overly critical of yourself if you weren't completely successful the first time—it can be a hard thing to do. Try to focus on what worked, why you think you slipped, and try again. Remember all of the reasons you want—and need—to quit smoking.

102. How soon will I start seeing the health benefits of not smoking?

There are some useful short-term and long-term benchmarks to help motivate you and keep you on the right track. For example,

- *Within several hours*, you will already start to realize some benefits of not smoking. For example, your heart rate and blood pressure will drop as nicotine leaves your system. Carbon monoxide from cigarette smoke—which binds to your red blood cells—will diminish to normal levels, allowing your red blood cells to carry more oxygen to your heart, brain, and the rest of your body.

- *Within two to three days*, your risk of heart attack will lessen and your senses of taste and smell will improve.

- *Within the first few weeks and months*, your circulation and tolerance for exercise and physical exertion will improve, and fatigue and shortness of breath will diminish.

- *A year after quitting smoking*, coronary heart disease risk is reduced by half.

103. I've heard that you always gain weight when you quit smoking. Is it inevitable?

It is common to gain a few pounds—perhaps between 6 and 10—for a while after you quit smoking, for a few reasons. Nicotine acts as an appetite suppressant, so quitting smoking will restore your normal appetite. Regular smoking can elevate your metabolism slightly, causing your body to burn a few extra calories. Finally, some people replace the habit of smoking with eating, so their daily calorie intake is increased. There are three things to remember to avoid using possible weight gain as an excuse to postpone quitting smoking:

- Even if you do gain a couple of pounds, the health benefits of quitting are life-changing—and maybe even life saving.

- For many people, the modest weight gain is temporary.
- Weight gain is not inevitable for everyone.

The simplest ways to minimize or avoid weight gain are, not surprisingly, to incorporate more exercise and physical activity into your daily routine, and to eat less food—and fewer high calorie foods. For example, when you snack instead of smoke, don't reach for the candy or cookies—try an apple, some carrots, or a 0% fat yogurt.

 PRACTICAL TIP To view the National Institute of Health's information on quitting smoking and weight gain, visit:

http://www.nih.gov/news/health/jun2011/nida-09.htm

If you have been diagnosed with heart disease, or have already had a heart attack or heart surgery, it is imperative that you quit smoking. There is a lot of readily available—and often free—information and support for you.

Managing Stress CHAPTER 18

104. How does stress contribute to heart disease?

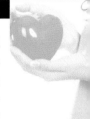

Most medical experts agree that emotional and psychological stress can be significant risk factors for heart disease, can worsen existing symptoms, and can increase the possibility of heart attack. While the complete cause-and-effect correlation between stress and heart disease is not entirely clear, the most commonly cited explanations include:

- Stress triggers our "fight or flight" reaction, which causes the release of stress hormones such as adrenaline and cortisol. Collectively, these hormones stimulate a number of significant effects on the body, such as constricting blood vessels, and raising heart rate, blood pressure, and blood sugar. They also affect the immune response and

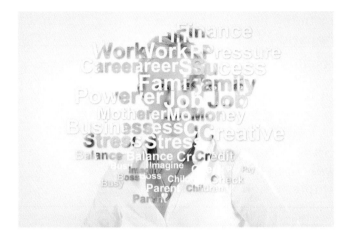

digestive system. This evolutionary physiological reaction to stress helps our bodies cope with threats, emergencies, and other temporary situations. But chronic stress can overload our systems with stress hormones and their effects, and interfere with our body's natural ability to return to its normal state.

- Stress may contribute to inflammation in the cardiovascular system, which is a significant factor in the development of atherosclerosis—the buildup of plaque in the coronary arteries.

- Our ways of coping with stress can increase several of the other major risk factors for heart disease, such as smoking, overeating and obesity, lack of exercise and physical activity, and alcohol and drug use.

105. Are there different kinds of stress?

Yes. Stress can result from countless daily annoyances, such as traffic jams, running late for work, spilling coffee on your clothes on the way out the door, or a barking dog when you're trying to sleep. On the other hand, stress can result from more significant circumstances that affect your psychological or emotional states in more constant and prolonged ways, such as your impaired health or that of a loved one, loss of a loved one, a demanding or frustrating career, personal relationship problems, or financial worries. Circumstances that cause you to feel stress and that trigger stress reactions are called *stressors*. Many stressors share the common characteristic of inflicting change on us, meaning that changed circumstances have altered our plans, routines, hopes, expectations, or beliefs. This requires us to react, change, and adapt—whether we want to or not—and creates stress.

We also experience a wide range of different emotional and psychological reactions to stressors. For example, we may feel angry, scared, hurt, or anxious, or we may experience more generalized—but more profound—feelings such as sadness, loneliness, or depression. Each of these emotions and feelings can trigger our body's physiological responses to stress, and jeopardize our heart health.

106. Does stress affect different people differently?

How different people perceive and react to stressful situations depends in large part on their psychological make-up—how each person is hard-wired. For example, what are often referred to as "Type A" people—those who prefer to be in control of circumstances, who may tend toward perfectionism, time sensitivity, and impatience, who are demanding of themselves and others—are more likely to have more intense stress reactions to daily annoyances and hassles. They may also experience more severe symptoms of stress as a result of the significant life circumstances that are stressful to everyone, like those we mentioned in Question 105. So-called Type B people—who tend to be more patient, low-key, and can better "roll with the punches"—are less likely to experience the same level of stress in nonurgent circumstances, and may have better coping mechanisms to moderate or manage their reaction to chronic stress. Not everyone fits into defined personality types or reacts to stress in predictable ways—the point is that people feel and react to stressors differently. Circumstances that may be very stressful for some people may not be at all stressful for others—they may be exciting. Some sports fans watching his or her team in the World

Series, or some parents watching a child in a recital or school play may feel stress, but that may also add to the experience. So yes—individual people react and respond differently to different types and levels of stress.

107. Isn't it normal to feel stress sometimes?

Feeling different types and levels of stress sometimes is completely normal, for two reasons. First, remember that our mind and body are programmed to recognize and react to stressful situations as part of our innate "fight or flight" system of self-preservation. Second, everyone's life includes situations and circumstances that produce stress. And stress is not always bad. For example, for some people stress can be a motivator, or add to the excitement of challenging circumstances. But what we're focusing on here is stress that can negatively affect your mind and body, and how to manage it to minimize its detrimental effects on your heart health.

108. How do I know whether the stress I'm feeling, and my reaction to it, is normal or unhealthy?

Experts cite a lengthy list of symptoms that can signal when someone's reaction to stress goes beyond normal to potentially unhealthy. Symptoms of stress can be categorized into three areas—physical, mental, and emotional. While temporarily experiencing one or two of these symptoms may not necessarily suggest a problem, if you find yourself fighting several symptoms, the symptoms last longer or are more severe than seems appropriate for the stressor, or the symptoms are interfering with your quality of life, or your ability to function to your fullest, talk with your doctor. Symptoms of stress can include:

- Muscle tension, aches and pains, clenching your jaw or fists, grinding your teeth, dizziness, or the feeling that your heart is racing
- Anger, hostility, or impatience
- Headaches, trouble sleeping, sleeping too much, or extreme fatigue

- Overeating, loss of appetite, or indigestion
- Inability to concentrate or forgetfulness
- Anxiety, crying, or irrational worry
- Sadness, depression, or feeling lonely or isolated
- Increased smoking, alcohol consumption, or drug use

109. How can I work to better cope with and manage my stress?

We could devote an entire book to this question alone. But for now, here are a number of strategies and techniques that may help you recognize your stressors and reduce the unhealthy effects that stress can have on your heart and cardiovascular system:

- Acknowledge that no one can eliminate all stress from his or her life. Some stress is both inevitable and normal. Don't create more stress by having unrealistic expectations!

- Be conscious of the situations and circumstances that are stressful for you. If you can avoid them, great—but that's not usually possible. However, you may be able to reduce some of them by saying "no" to additional demands or expectations and exercising more control over your schedule and priorities.

- Set aside time to relax each day, even if only for a short time. Read, listen to music, cook, watch TV, work in your garden, chat with a friend or family member (who doesn't create stress)—whatever calms you and restores your internal sense of balance.

- Explore physical relaxation techniques, such as:
  - Deep breathing exercises
  - Meditation
  - Yoga
  - Taking a walk
  - Getting a massage

- Get regular exercise.
- Eat regular meals of healthy foods. Avoid too much coffee—caffeine is a stimulant.
- Shorten your "to-do list."
- Have someone you trust to talk to. Sometimes simply talking through stressful situations can help you moderate your anxiety.
- Get plenty of sleep. If chronic sleeplessness is one of your symptoms of stress, talk to your doctor about whether a prescription or over-the-counter sleep aid might be appropriate.
- Avoid smoking and overuse of alcohol. While many smokers feel that smoking relieves stress, in fact nicotine is a stimulant that can exacerbate your reaction to stress. Similarly, while a small amount of alcohol may provide temporary feelings of relaxation, excessive alcohol consumption can reduce your ability to cope with stress—in addition to creating other health risks.
- Think positive. For example, take a reasoned approach to short-term stressors, such as reminding yourself that a particular situation is not worth getting so worked up over, or remind yourself that your short-term stressors will resolve quickly. Try breaking down seemingly overwhelming stressors into smaller pieces that you can manage if you're flexible. Give yourself credit for your successes rather than dwell on things you wish you had done differently or better. Work to solve the situations you know you can solve, rather than get consumed with those you can't. Finally, acknowledge that there are some things you just cannot control, or the outcome may be undesirable, and that some situations or circumstances might always be hard or painful. One coping strategy might be to work on keeping long-term and irresolvable stressors in a mental "box" separate from the parts of your life

that give you pleasure, fulfill you, sustain you, and nourish you. Allow yourself the time and space to tackle the toughest challenges on *your* terms.

If, in spite of your best efforts, stress continues to dominate your thoughts, feelings, and behavior, talk to your doctor. He or she may recommend trying prescription medication, or a referral to a mental health professional because keeping undue stress at bay is critical to maintaining your heart health.

CASE STUDY

While stress alone is a significant risk factor for heart disease, a lifestyle that creates stress can also contribute to other risk factors as well. Consider Beth's experience.

Beth is a successful businesswoman in her early 50s who is under constant pressure to cultivate clients— and their revenue. As always, it seemed, she was running late for an important meeting and stuck in heavy traffic. In her own words, she was getting very agitated because the meeting was in one hour and she knew she wouldn't make it. As she grew more stressed about the traffic jam, Beth suddenly began to feel unwell, with pain in her chest that travelled to her shoulder and down her arm. She thought she had a cramp, but then became very hot and short of breath. With traffic at a standstill, she opened her car door and collapsed in the road unconscious.

Beth was lucky in two respects. A nurse was in a nearby car, and ran over to help. The nurse instructed a bystander to call 911, and, with the aid of another driver, started cardiopulmonary resuscitation (CPR). The road Beth was travelling on had a breakdown lane that allowed the ambulance to get to her quickly, give her oxygen and medication, and take her to the hospital. The speed of everyone's response likely saved her life. She regained consciousness at the hospital. When tests revealed she had suffered a moderate heart attack, Beth expressed a number of thoughts that everyone can learn from.

Beth considered herself reasonably fit, was not overweight, and believed that men got heart disease—rarely women. She never thought she could be at risk for a heart attack. But tests revealed that Beth's hard-driving and stressful work demands resulted in a number of significant heart disease risks that had gone undetected because she never took time for regular check-ups:

- High blood pressure
- High cholesterol
- Sedentary lifestyle and lack of exercise

The stress of being stuck in traffic on the way to an important meeting may have been the final trigger for Beth's heart attack, but it wasn't the cause. It was the constant stress in her life that exposed Beth to several of the highest risk factors for heart disease. Beth was lucky and has recovered. She gets regular exercise, takes cholesterol medication, and has left her stressful job for part-time work. And she's more relaxed, happier, and in control of her heart health.

Adapted from CardiacMatters

Diet and Nutrition

110. How does diet affect cardiovascular health?

We mentioned in Part Two some of the reasons why unhealthy dietary habits are significant contributors to heart disease. For example, poor diet can cause obesity and related high blood pressure and place undue strain on the heart. Poor diet is a primary cause of atherosclerosis—the accumulation of dangerous plaque in the coronary arteries—as a result of high harmful fat and cholesterol levels. In this chapter, we're going to take a closer look at these and some of the other key dietary factors that can affect your cardiovascular health.

111. I know I shouldn't eat too much, but how much should I be eating?

Before we go into how much of certain *kinds* of food we should eat or avoid, let's first talk about total daily calorie intake. Remember that a calorie is a unit of energy. All food you eat contains calories, which are either used by the body for the countless functions that require energy, or the calories are stored—typically as fat on the body. Calorie intake is determined by how much you eat of different types of foods, because different foods have different calorie content. Carbohydrates and protein contain four calories per gram, while fat contains nine calories per gram. Recommended daily calorie intake can vary significantly depending on a person's age, sex, and level of activity. For example, the United States Department of Agriculture and Department of Health and Human Services dietary guidelines suggest three levels of daily calorie intake:

- About 1600 calories/day for very young children, most women, and some older adults
- About 2200 calories/day for older children, teenage girls, active women, and most men
- About 2800 calories/day for teenage boys and active men

The calorie intake guidelines are just that—guidelines. Not everyone within a category will have the same calorie needs to maintain good health as other people in that category, and each person's calorie needs change depending on their level of activity on any given day. But the guidelines serve as a good benchmark as you plan your diet.

To make the calorie guidelines useful and practical for people to plan and manage healthy diet and nutrition habits, they are converted into servings of food from different food groups based on the nutritional content of each group. We'll talk about specific food content and nutrition shortly.

112. What are some simple ways to avoid eating too much?

The two primary dietary causes for obesity are eating too much, and eating too many high calorie, low nutrition foods. Here are some ways to manage your food intake:

- *Control your portion size.* Put the least amount of food on your plate that you might reasonably eat. Load up on low calorie foods such as vegetables, and keep portions of high calorie foods smaller. Dietary guidelines for healthy eating have specific serving or portion sizes. For example, according to the United States Department of Agriculture (USDA), one serving of cooked pasta is ½ cup, and one serving of a raw leafy vegetable is one cup. The USDA recognizes that you may eat more than one serving of a certain food at a meal, so you would estimate how many servings you ate. Because a healthy diet will include multiple servings from each food group every day, eating

Pay attention to serving sizes of packaged products—they have gotten bigger over the years because it's more profitable for the companies that sell them. For example, a soft drink (and we're not advocating drinking high-sugar soda) used to come only in 12 oz. cans. In fact, Coca-Cola® was originally sold in their famous 6 oz. bottles. But most soft drinks are now sold in 20 oz. bottles. Don't let commercial packaging dictate how much you consume.

PRACTICAL TIP

more than one serving at a meal is fine, as long as you don't eat more than necessary at any one meal.

- *Eat slowly.* Your body releases hormones in response to food and liquid in the stomach as a signal that you're getting full, but it can take up to twenty minutes for the brain to get this message. Until then, you still feel hungry. If you eat too quickly, you may eat more food than you need because you haven't given your body time to respond to the "full" signal.

- *Drink water with your meal.* Water will both make you feel more full, and help slow your eating. Water also aids in digestion.

- *Hold off on a second helping.* Give your body time to react to what you've already eaten. You'll likely find that you don't really *need* the second plateful. If the food is that delicious, save the rest for a meal the next day.

- *Munch on healthy snacks during the day.* The old saying "don't eat before dinner because it will spoil your appetite" doesn't promote healthy eating habits. Over the course of a day, most people will consume fewer calories if they munch on nutritious snacks when they feel hungry. Healthy snacking promotes a regular supply of the nutrients your body needs, and helps stave off a ravenous appetite at mealtime that often leads to hurried overeating.

- *Avoid eating meals in front of the TV.* Eating meals while watching television can cause you to eat faster, and to eat more because you're distracted from how much you're eating.

- *Avoid eating late at night.* Your body doesn't need lots of calories right before sleeping, so if you feel hungry because dinner was several hours ago, drink a glass of water, or have a cup of tea. Some research shows that green tea in particular may act as a mild appetite suppressant, and the water will help you feel full.

113. What foods should I should I eat more of? What foods should I avoid?

There are many different ways to categorize foods as we think about planning a heart-healthy diet. In fact, after undergoing a series of revisions over the years, the government's iconic "food pyramid" was replaced in 2011 by the United States Department of Agriculture with a new concept of food groups and servings called MyPlate:

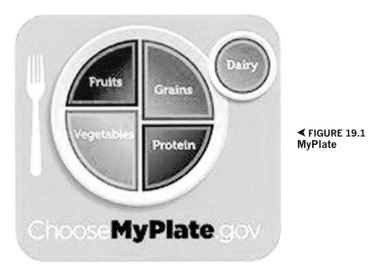

◀ FIGURE 19.1
MyPlate

SOURCE: http://www.choosemyplate.gov/images/MyPlateImages/PDF/myplate_green.pdf

To read about the Department of Agriculture's MyPlate concept, accompanying description of food groups, and recommended foods and serving sizes within each group, visit:

http://www.choosemyplate.gov/food-groups/

MyPlate is divided into 5 categories of food:

- Dairy
- Vegetables
- Fruits

- Grains
- Protein

However, rather than discuss each of the categories on MyPlate, we're going to focus on the aspects of diet and nutrition that have the greatest impact on cardiovascular health.

114. What do I need to know about fats and oils?

The recently replaced food pyramid—which is still accepted as a reference point—indicated that we should consume from the fats and oils group "sparingly." There are two main types of bad dietary fats that contribute to heart disease— saturated fat and trans fats. As we've touched on earlier, these fats can raise LDL (bad) cholesterol levels and are often found in foods that are already high in LDL cholesterol. They may also lower your HDL (good) cholesterol. Each of these factors contributes to atherosclerosis—the buildup of plaque in the coronary arteries which is the leading cause of heart disease and the primary precursor to heart attack. And as we noted in Question 111, all fats contain the most calories per gram of any of our food sources, so it can be a significant contributor to unhealthy weight.

However, not all fats and oils are the same—in moderation, some are good for our heart and cardiovascular health because they may raise HDL (good) cholesterol, may help lower LDL cholesterol, and contain essential fatty acids that are a necessary part of our diet. Unsaturated fats are in this category. So when you do consume or cook with foods with high fat and oil content, avoid the bad ones. Examples of foods high in bad fats include:

- Butter, cheese, and ice cream.
- Red meat, and fattier cuts of any meat and poultry.
- Coconut and palm oil; cocoa butter.
- Foods fried in saturated fat, such as french fries and doughnuts.

- Commercially baked goods, such as cookies, crackers, pizza, muffins, and pastries. These often contain "trans fat" which is a manufactured fat also known as "partially hydrogenated oils." Trans fats are used because they add to the flavor, texture, and shelf life of these products. The Food and Drug Administration requires commercially prepared foods to list the unsaturated, saturated, and trans fat content on the Nutrition Facts label, so check before you buy. The American Heart Association recommends that most people limit their consumption of saturated fats to about 7% of your daily calorie intake, and limit trans fats to 1%.

> **PRACTICAL TIP**
>
> Using the American Heart Association's 7% and 1% guidelines, if you are on a 2000 calories per day diet, that would mean limiting your consumption of saturated fats to 140 calories, and trans fat to 20 calories. At 9 calories per gram of fat, that equates to about 16 grams of saturated fat and less than 2 grams of trans fat.

Examples of foods high in good fat and oil (unsaturated fat) include:

- Vegetable oils, such as olive oil, canola oil, sunflower oil, sesame oil, peanut oil, soybean oil, and corn oil.
- Many seeds and nuts, such as flaxseed, almonds, peanuts (great news for peanut butter lovers!), walnuts, sunflower seeds; avocados.
- Fattier fish, such as salmon, herring, trout, tuna, and mackerel. The key benefit of these fish—especially salmon and herring—is that their fat contains a fatty acid called "omega-3." Omega-3 fatty acids are a type of unsaturated fat that research suggests may be particularly effective in promoting cardiovascular health by reducing triglycerides, boosting HDL cholesterol, lowering LDL cholesterol, reducing vascular inflammation, and lowering blood pressure. Eating at least two servings of high-omega-3 fish per week is believed to have a beneficial effect on heart health.

Remember that while the good fats and oils can contribute to your heart and cardiovascular health, they are still calorie heavy. The American Heart Association recommends that we limit our total consumption of fat to 25%–35% of our total calories each day. For someone on a 2000 calorie per day diet, this means 500–700 calories from fat, or 55–77 grams of fat.

 For a personalized Body Mass Index assessment and caloric intake recommendations, try the American Heart Association's *My Fat Translator*:

http://www.heart.org/HEARTORG/
GettingHealthy/FatsAndOils/Fats101/
My-Fats-Translator_UCM_428869_
Article.jsp

By comparison, the USDA's MyPlate suggests a certain "allowance" of oil per day, based on age, sex, and activity level. For example, for men over 30 who get regular exercise the allowance is six teaspoons, and for women over 30 the allowance is five teaspoons. To see what constitutes a teaspoon of oil in a variety of common foods with high oil content, visit:
http://www.ChooseMyPlate.gov/food-groups/oils-count.
html#

CASE STUDY

In the mid-1990s, a long-term study—called the Women's Health Initiative Dietary Modification Trial—undertook to examine the effects of dietary modification on almost 49,000 post-menopausal women of diverse backgrounds and ethnicities. Specifically, the Trial sought to examine the influence of a reduced fat diet on breast cancer, and secondarily its influence on cardiovascular disease. To achieve the desired behavior modification, the test group was given initial and on-going nutritional education on how to reduce total fat to 20% of daily caloric intake, increase servings of fruits and vegetables to five per day, and increase servings of grains to six per day.

The Trial did not specifically instruct participants to distinguish among saturated, unsaturated, or trans fat in the diet. Each participant was given a personal fat intake goal based on her height. Participants were surveyed every six months on diet, exercise, and health changes, given physical examinations annually, and underwent an EKG every three years. Medical issues relating to cardiovascular health (angina, diagnosis of cardiovascular disease, heart attacks) were recorded.

The participants were followed for an average of about eight years. As a group, they achieved only an 8.2% reduction in daily caloric fat intake (versus the target of 20%), and modest increases in daily servings of fruits, vegetables, and grains. While the details of the study and analysis of the results are lengthy and complex, there were a few key findings worth noting for our discussion. The trial group experienced:

- A small decrease in LDL (bad) cholesterol
- A small decrease in diastolic blood pressure
- Decreases in weight and waist size
- No measurable decrease in cardiovascular disease as a group, BUT:
- The participants who reduced their intake of saturated fat and trans fat by the greatest amounts had a lower incidence of cardiovascular disease

The Trial concluded that a modest reduction in both good and bad fats and modest increase in fruits, vegetables, and grains may not have a direct impact on the incidence of cardiovascular disease. Most importantly, however, there was sufficient evidence to suggest that replacing bad fats with good fats, and increasing consumption of fruits, vegetables, and grains did show a correlation to reduced cardiovascular disease.

DEFINITION Simply stated, **carbohydrates** are substances built on sugar molecules. The scientific structure of different carbohydrates is varied and complex, but our most common dietary carbohydrates fall into one of three categories—simple carbohydrates, complex carbohydrates, and fiber. The classification is determined by the number and structure of sugar molecules.

Sugar is the main source of our body's energy, and carbohydrates contribute the most calories to our diet—anywhere from 40%–65% of our daily caloric intake. The nutritional value of carbohydrate sources varies among the three categories. Let's take a look at types of carbohydrates, how they contribute to our nutrition and health, and examples of foods in each category.

- *Simple carbohydrates.* In general, simple carbohydrates are those with one or two chains of sugar molecules. The body quickly metabolizes simple carbohydrates into glucose, the usable form of sugar. While all carbohydrates provide energy when the body converts them to glucose, some foods that contain simple carbohydrates are healthy primarily because of other, non-carbohydrate nutrients they contain that are necessary for our overall health. These include:

  — Milk products (preferably low or no fat), which in addition to containing the simple sugars galactose and lactose, contribute protein, minerals, and vitamins to our diet.

  — Fruits, which contain the simple sugar fructose, but also contain vitamins, minerals, and fiber.

- Vegetables, some of which contain the simple sugar maltose (as does beer), but which also contain vitamins, minerals, fiber, and in some cases, protein.

On the other hand, many foods containing large amounts of simple sugars have little nutritional value, can overload our body with glucose (see Question 116 concerning glycemic index), and therefore increase our risk for weight gain and diabetes. Examples include:

- Soda, sports drinks, and refined fruit juices—though some are supplemented with vitamins and minerals.
- Candy, cookies, and similar snack foods.

These types of foods not only lack nutrients essential for cardiovascular health, they make you feel full and keep you from eating foods that are good for your heart. If you've heard the term "empty calories," it refers to the foods in this group that are high sugar, high calorie, low nutrition foods that are some of the worst culprits for unhealthy weight gain.

- *Complex carbohydrates.* Complex carbohydrates are those with three or more chains of sugars. Foods we commonly think of as "starch" fall into this category. Because of their higher complexity, many compound carbohydrates take longer for the body to break down and help you feel fuller for a longer period of time. Among other benefits, this controls hunger and overeating—and therefore helps with weight management. Equally important, foods high in complex carbohydrates typically contain other nutrients essential to heart health. However, not all complex carbohydrates are equally heart-healthy. Many common foods are complex carbohydrates as a matter of chemical structure, but are metabolized by the body quickly, and therefore have effects on our body more resembling simple carbohydrates. Examples include:

- Highly processed grains, such as white flour, which is used in common foods such as white bread, processed cereals, and white pasta.
- Potatoes and white rice.

While these foods have some nutritional value, there are much heart-healthier foods to build the carbohydrate portion of your diet, including:

- Whole, unrefined grains such as wheat, barley, and rye.
- Fruits and vegetables, which in addition contain some simple carbohydrates, also contain complex forms.
- Legumes (a sub-category of vegetables), such as beans, lentils, and peas.

- *Fiber.* Fiber is an indigestible form of carbohydrate. There are two types—soluble and insoluble—and most high-fiber foods contain both. Soluble fiber is believed to contribute to your cardiovascular health in a number of ways, including:
  - Helping you feel full and reducing overeating,
  - Lowering LDL (bad) cholesterol, thereby reducing the build up of plaque in the coronary arteries,
  - Lowering blood pressure, and
  - Controlling blood sugar levels.

There are many foods that contain both fiber and other essential nutrients like protein, vitamins, minerals, and complex carbohydrates, but a few examples include:

- Fruits (especially with the skin) and vegetables
- Whole grains
- Bran
- Legumes

To eat healthier, go for color—a colorful plate is heart-healthy one!

HEART HEALTH

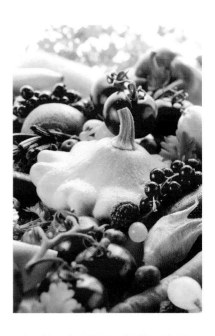

116. What is the "glycemic index" and "glycemic load"?

Some recent research into diet and health suggests that in addition to a correlation between high bad cholesterol, triglycerides, and heart disease, there is growing evidence of a high correlation between volatile blood sugar levels and heart disease. A food's *glycemic index* typically refers to how quickly the body converts the carbohydrates in the food to glucose and gets it into the blood. A high glycemic index food raises blood glucose quickly, while a low glycemic index food results in a more moderated effect on blood glucose. Glycemic index is measured on a scale of 1–100, and following are examples of the glycemic index of some common foods:

GLYCEMIC INDEX RANGE	FOOD (AVERAGE SERVING)
High (70 and higher)	White rice, white bread, baked potato, watermelon
Medium (56–69)	Corn, raisins, banana
Low (55 and under)	Skim milk, raw carrots, peanuts, lentils, kidney beans

Some foods, like watermelon, have a high glycemic index because the sugar is quickly converted to glucose in the blood. However, since watermelon is mostly water, the sugar content is not that high, so while the sugar is converted to glucose quickly, there isn't that much if it. To more accurately account for the impact of a food on blood sugar, experts use the concept of *glycemic load.*

Glycemic load takes into account both the speed with which a food's sugar is converted to glucose, as well as how much glucose is produced by factoring in sugar content and portion size. Glycemic load gives a better assessment of the negative impact of a food on our body. Ranges of glycemic loads are High (20 and higher), Medium (11–19), and Low (10 and under). Not surprisingly, foods with high amounts of simple sugars—soda, candy, cake, and doughnuts, for example—and some foods with high amounts of quickly converted complex sugars— like potatoes—have a high glycemic load. And to give you an idea of the difference between processed and unprocessed foods, regular oatmeal has a glycemic index

To see the Harvard Medical School's *Glycemic Index and Glycemic Load for 100+ Foods,* visit:

http://www.health.harvard.edu/ newsweek/Glycemic_index_and_ glycemic_load_for_100_foods.htm

of 55 (low) and a glycemic load of 13 (medium), while instant oatmeal has a glycemic index of 83 (high) and a glycemic load of 30 (high)!

Why is all of this important to cardiovascular health? Because rapid spikes in blood sugar cause the body to produce more of the hormone insulin, which instructs the body's cells to take in glucose from the bloodstream. A constant diet of high glycemic load foods is believed to be a significant risk factor for heart disease because:

- Constant, extreme reactions to blood glucose can overwork the body's capacity to make—and stop making—insulin as blood sugar rises and falls quickly. This can cause a condition known as insulin resistance, and raises the risk of developing diabetes.
- Sugar that cannot be used by the body is stored as fat, and can lead to obesity.
- There is also evidence that rapid spikes in blood sugar can contribute to inflammation of the cardiovascular system, which in turn contributes to atherosclerosis—plaque in the arteries.
- High glycemic load foods can contribute to high blood pressure.

Studies have shown that women have a stronger correlation between high glycemic load diets and heart disease than men do.

NOTE

HEART HEALTH

To see the Harvard School of Public Health's five tips for adding good carbs to your diet, visit:

http://www.hsph.harvard.edu/ nutritionsource/what-should-you-eat/ carbohydrates/

The food groups that we have already mentioned—often called the "good carbs" such as fruits, vegetables, legumes, nuts, and whole grains—typically have lower glycemic loads than the "bad carb" foods. While not all medical professionals and nutrition experts agree on the role and significance of glycemic index and glycemic load in cardiovascular health compared to other risk factors, the impact of high glycemic load food on the body's metabolism seems clear.

Hopefully you see a clear pattern here of the types of foods that should form the basis of your heart-healthy diet—and those to avoid. You don't need to spend a lot of time understanding the technical science of nutrition and heart health to put it into practice. And one final note: everyone has a favorite snack or dessert that may not make the list of healthiest foods. That's OK. No one would suggest giving up entirely an occasional treat. As long as your balanced diet favors foods with good fats and good carbs, you'll be well on your way to a healthy heart!

 You can look up the calorie, protein, and good and bad fat content of over 1200 common foods in the United States Department of Agriculture's Nutritive Value of Foods at:

http://www.ars.usda.gov/SP2UserFiles/Place/12354500/Data/hg72/hg72_2002.pdf

Index

A

ACE. *See* angiotensin converting
    enzyme
aerobic exercise
    for cardiovascular health, 42–43
    definition, 41–42
alpha blockers, 94
American Heart Association, 24, 33,
    120–121
anaerobic exercise, 42
anemia, 10
angina
    case study, 62–63
    common medications, 51
    definition, 48
    other conditions, 51–52
    other indications, 52
    stable, 49
    treatment, 50–51
    types, 49–50
    unstable, 49
    variant, 49–50
angina pectoris. *See* angina
angioplasty procedures, 77–78
angiotensin converting enzyme
    (ACE), 94
angiotensin II receptor blockers
    (ARBs), 94
antiarrhythmia drugs, 96–97
anti-coagulants, 71
anti-platelet drugs, 70
apolipoproteins (Apos), 61
ARBs. *See* angiotensin II receptor
    blockers
arrhythmias, 83, 96
arterioles, 7
atherosclerosis, 15, 64

B

"bad carbs," 128
bad cholesterol. *See* low-density
    lipoproteins (LDL)
    cholesterol
beta blockers, 51, 94
bile acid sequestrants, 92–93
biventricular pacemaker, 83
blood
    components
      plasma, 9
      platelets, 10–11
      red blood cells, 9–10

white blood cells, 10
    flow through heart, 5–6
blood pressure
    definition, 27
    measurement, 28
    for men and women, 29–30
    numbers, 28–29
blood pressure drugs
    alpha blockers, 94
    angiotensin converting enzyme, 94
    angiotensin II receptor blockers, 94
    beta blockers, 94
    calcium channel blockers, 94–95
    diuretics, 95
    renin inhibitors, 95
    vasodilators, 95
blood tests
    coronary heart disease, 59–61
    heart attack, 68–70
    heart failure, 61
blood thinners, 70, 96
BMI. *See* body mass index
BNPs. *See* B-type natriuretic
    peptides
body mass index (BMI)
    control, 37–38
    definition, 34
    interpretation, 36
    measurement, 35–36
bradycardia, 83
B-type natriuretic peptides (BNPs), 61

C

CAIs. *See* cholesterol absorption
    inhibitors
calcium channel blockers, 51, 94–95
capillaries, 7
carbohydrates
    complex, 124–125
    definition, 123
    fiber, 125
    simple, 123–124
cardiac rehabilitation
    definition, 88–89
    importance, 89
cardiac resynchronization therapy, 83
cardiac stress test, 54
cardiovascular system
    definition, 6
    working system, 8
CAT. *See* computed axial tomography

CDC. *See* Centers for Disease Control and Prevention
CECs. *See* circulating endothelial cells
Centers for Disease Control and Prevention (CDC), 14, 16, 65, 71
CHD. *See* coronary heart disease
chest X-ray, 55
cholesterol
  definition, 17–18
  diet, 21–23
  drug therapies
    bile acid sequestrants, 92–93
    cholesterol absorption inhibitors, 93
    fibrates, 93
    niacin, 92
    statins, 90–92
  factors affecting, 20
  healthy levels, 18–20
  high-density lipoproteins, 18–20
  low-density lipoproteins, 18–19
  regular exercise, 21
  total, 18–19
cholesterol absorption inhibitors (CAIs), 93
circulating endothelial cells (CECs), 62
CKP. *See* creatine phosphokinase
"clot busting" drugs, 70
clot preventing drugs, 70
complex carbohydrates, 124–125
computed axial tomography (CAT), 57
congestive heart failure, 37
coronary angiogram, 56
coronary angioplasty, 71
coronary arteries, 7
coronary artery bypass grafting (CABG), 78
coronary bypass, 78
coronary bypass surgery
  other types, 80
  procedures, 78–79
  recovery process, 81–82
  risks, 80–81
coronary heart disease (CHD)
  affecting heart, 15–16
  case study, 62–63
  causes, 15
  definition, 14
  diagnostic procedures

    blood tests, 59–61
    cardiac stress test, 54
    chest X-ray, 55
    computed axial tomography, 57
    coronary angiogram, 56
    echocardiogram, 54–55
    electrocardiogram, 53–54
    Holter monitor, 58
    magnetic resonance imaging, 57
    positron emission tomography, 58
  pacemakers, 82–83
  prescribed drugs, 89–90
  prevalent factors, 100
  risk factors, 16–17
  signs and symptoms, 48
C-reactive protein (CRP), 59–60
creatine phosphokinase (CKP), 69
CRP. *See* C-reactive protein

D

diabetes
  definition, 33
  risk factor for heart disease, 33–34
diagnostic procedures
  blood tests, 59–61
  cardiac stress test, 54
  chest X-ray, 55
  computed axial tomography, 57
  coronary angiogram, 56
  echocardiogram, 54–55
  electrocardiogram, 53–54
  Holter monitor, 58
  magnetic resonance imaging, 57
  positron emission tomography, 58
diastolic pressure, 28
diet
  affecting cardiovascular health, 115
  affecting cholesterol levels, 21–23
  calorie intake, 115–116
  case study, 121–122
  fats and oils, 119–121
  managing food intake, 116–117
  MyPlate concept, 118–119
diuretics, 95
drug-eluting stents, 75

E

echocardiogram, 54–55
EKG. *See* electrocardiogram
electrocardiogram (EKG), 53–54

O

obesity
 causes, 36
 definition, 34
 risk factor for heart disease, 37
off-pump bypass surgery, 80
Omega-3 fatty acids, 26
on-pump bypass surgery, 79

P

pacemaker, 82–83
partial hydrogenation, 23–24
pericardium, 4
PET. *See* positron emission
  tomography
plasma, 9
platelets, 10–11
positron emission tomography
  (PET), 58
post-traumatic stress disorder
  (PTSD), 87
primary hypertension, 30–31
Prinzmetal's angina, 49–50
PTSD. *See* post-traumatic stress
  disorder

R

red blood cells, 9–10
regular exercise, 21
renin inhibitors, 95

S

saturated fat, 23
secondary hypertension, 31
simple carbohydrates, 123–124
smokeless tobacco, 40
smoking
 quitting
  description, 39
  hard to, 102
  health benefits, 106
  reasons, 101–102
  slip and smoke, 105
  strategies, 102–104
  weight gain, 106–107
  withdrawal, 105
 risk factor for heart disease, 38
soluble fiber, 125
sphygmomanometer, 28
stable angina, 49

statins, 90–92
stress
 affecting people, 109–110
 case study, 113–114
 for heart disease, 107–108
 normal, 110
 symptoms, 110–111
 types, 108–109
 unhealthy effects, 111–113
stressors, 109
systolic pressure, 28

T

tachycardia, 83
"the silent killer." *See* high
  blood pressure
thrombocytes, 10–11
thrombolytics, 70
tobacco, smokeless, 40
tomography
 computed axial, 57
 definition, 56–57
 magnetic resonance imaging, 57
 positron emission, 58
total cholesterol, 18–19
transfat, 23–24
transfatty acids, 23–24
triglycerides
 definition, 18, 24
 healthy levels, 24–25
 risk factor for heart disease, 24
troponin test, 69
type 1 diabetes, 33
type 2 diabetes, 33

U

United States Department of
  Agriculture (USDA), 115–116,
  118, 121
unsaturated fat, 24
unstable angina, 49
USDA. *See* United States
  Department of Agriculture

V

variant angina, 49–50
vasodilators, 95

W

white blood cells, 10